HOW TO FIGHT
PROSTATE CANCER AND WIN

Advice On:

Natural Prevention

Alternative Self-treatments

Medical Testing

Therapeutic Diets

William L. Fischer

AGORA HEALTH BOOKS
BALTIMORE, MARYLAND

How to Fight
Prostate Cancer and Win

How to Fight Prostate Cancer and Win

A Practical Guide to Prostate Health

ISBN 1-891434-09-8

Printed in England

AGORA HEALTH BOOKS
819 N. Charles St.
Baltimore, MD 21201
www.thehealthierlife.co.uk

TABLE OF CONTENTS

P R E F A C E

Prostate disorders of some form, statistics tell us, will affect the average man over age 40 sometime during his life. One in every eight men will develop prostate cancer in their lifetime. Moreover, approximately 180,000 will develop prostate cancer this year alone. Pretty scary facts.

But these figures aren't etched in stone. The average man can reduce his chances of developing prostate cancer and other prostate problems with some simple, common-sense steps.

This is the objective of this book—to help men prevent prostate problems and cancer. For those who are quietly suffering with these conditions, the goal is to find ways to relieve the pain.

The reader will find diagnostic and treatment methods used by modern medicine outlined here, as well as several prostate relievers and cures that lie outside the medical mainstream.

Nutritional research is finding that the key to a lifetime free of prostate troubles is lying on your dinner plate—or should be. A proper diet, plus several nutritional supplements, can help men avoid and alleviate prostate ailments.

Exercise is also an important part of keeping the gland free of prostatitis or prostatic hypertrophy well into a man's golden years. This updated and fully revised edition of *How to Fight Prostate Cancer and Win* explains which exercises are the best and why. In fact, this book provides invaluable insight into natural ways of staying healthy and having prostate problems solved before they manifest themselves.

The same prescription applies to men who want to avoid prostate cancer. I have included instructions for an important self-examination for detecting testicular cancer.

It is not a widely known disease, but it is deadly if not discovered in time.

The delicate subject of impotency is examined with honesty and sensitivity, in language easy for the layman to understand. It offers hope through natural methods as well as new remedies only recently obtainable in the United States.

This book deserves the attention of every man—and of any woman concerned about the well-being of her male loved ones. It demystifies the prostate gland and provides hope to those who suffer from impotency. It is hoped that this updated edition of *How to Fight Prostate Cancer and Win* will be a friend wherever it goes; that it will help you to return to nature's way of caring for your body.

William L. Fischer

COMMENTS and REVIEWS for
How to Fight Prostate Cancer and Win.

J. Orsini, athletic trainer, UCLA
former National Weightlifting Champion:

"As a sports figure and health expert, I found William Fischer's book *[How to Fight Prostate Cancer and Win]** to be a jewel. Not only did I find the advice concerning the prostate gland and impotency to be sound, but I recommended the book to several of my friends. These older gentlemen were all suffering from some type of prostate problem.

They were relieved to read a book that understood their pain and were delighted when they put the advice into practice. Between the natural products, such as flower pollen extract and kombucha, and the dietary guidelines (important for every man to read, regardless of his age or the state of his prostate), each of my friends found a method or combination of methods that alleviated his problem. None of them suffers any longer—thanks to William Fischer's *[How to Fight Prostate Cancer and Win]**.

This may just be the most important book you read this year. It contains life-saving information that can change the way you live. I'm sure you will find this book to be as informative as I did, and I am equally sure that the suggestions and recommendations can help your prostate disorders as effectively as they did those of my friends.

[How to Fight Prostate Cancer and Win]'s* practical approach to problems that so many face is most welcome. This book is a necessary addition to any home medical library."

E. Groth, N.D.
Naturopathic physician:

"Exhaustively researched, very well-written, filled with life-saving information: a gold mine of advice and suggestions."These were my impressions of William Fischer's latest book, *[How to Fight Prostate Cancer and Win]**. He has succeeded in producing an intelligently written and highly sensitive volume on a topic not easily spoken of— the prostate and its effect on a man's emotional and physical health.

At long last, the public has a book it deserves on a subject too long neglected. *[How to Fight Prostate Cancer and Win]** explains why the tiny prostate gland looms so large in the health of men— especially men in their 40s and beyond.

This book is a keeper, to be read over and over again and used as a reference. Its advice is not only easy to implement but inexpensive as well. It outlines modern medical techniques while showing low-cost alternative methods to achieving good health.

Ladies cannot afford to ignore this book, either—so packed is it with information vital to their own health and happiness."

C.H., a prostate patient:

"Several years ago I developed some problems with my prostate gland. The troubles looked innocent enough at first, but they eventually grew and the situation got more serious.

Someone loaned me a copy of *[How to Fight Prostate Cancer and Win]**. I have to admit that I was skeptical at first. Nontheless, I started off with some of your suggestions. Well, before I knew it, my problem had eased up. My doctor surely was surprised ("shocked" would be a better word) and I made sure I always checked with him every so often. Like I said, I was skeptical.

My prostate problems are gone, I'm happier than I've ever been and, believe it or not, I feel I have the energy of someone half my age! Bless you!"

C.C.N., *prostate patient:*

"The doctor told me only surgery would help my problem. Naturally, I was reluctant to undergo a prostate operation.

I bought the book *[How to Fight Prostate Cancer and Win]** and learned there were sound natural alternatives to surgery. I immediately put your advice into use. My wife made fun of me at first, but she's not laughing now!

Just last week, my doctor told me the inflammation was so slight that the operation would not be needed. What a wonderful alternative to surgery! And, by the way, after following some of your advice on diet and exercise, I feel years younger. I think I may have found myself a new life."

F.Z., *prostate patient:*

"At 67, I developed a prostate problem. My friends told me it was a natural part of aging.

I picked up your book and was astonished to learn that even at my age I can avoid these problems. I bought some of those natural products you mentioned in the book and started eating better. My wife and I started walking every day.

You guessed it! I haven't had any more problems. For me, it really was a *[How to Fight Prostate Cancer and Win]**.

I bought a copy for my son, who is in his early 40s. Maybe he can avoid prostate problems altogether."

Mrs. A.F.C., wife of a prostate patient:

"I can't thank you enough for your book [How to Fight Prostate Cancer and Win]*. My husband had suffered from impotency for quite a while but was too embarrassed to seek medical help. I bought your book and read it myself.

Imagine my surprise when I discovered that some prescription drugs can cause impotency! The medication my husband was taking appeared in your book. I showed this to him, and he finally agreed to talk with his doctor. The doctor was only too happy to change his prescription.

Today, we are enjoying a truly loving marriage. Thank you so much.

By the way, my husband showed your book to the doctor, who thought it was very good, extremely well-researched, and of great benefit."

J.C.B., prostatitis patient:

I'm not a health expert or any type of nutritional specialist. I am just an average guy—a guy who used to suffer from prostatitis.

But thanks to William Fischer's latest book, [How to Fight Prostate Cancer and Win]*, I no longer am bothered by my prostate. I spent literally years searching for a doctor who could help me, but I found no relief. Finally, I gave up and resigned myself to living with the pain.

My wife bought me a copy of [How to Fight Prostate Cancer and Win]*, but I was sure it would be of no use to me. Boy, was I wrong! There was so much sound advice. I can't imagine any man's not finding something that agrees with his body and his lifestyle. I was thrilled to discover that two products worked especially well for me. The answer to my problem was so simple."

* Formerly titled *Miraculous Breakthroughs for Prostate and Impoteny Problems.*

• C H A P T E R 1 •

What Is a Prostate Gland?

The male prostate gland weighs barely an ounce and is only the size of a walnut, but it has a great effect on the male reproductive system—and the self-images of thousands of men who feel its less-than-positive effects as their years add up.

The prostate gland is a doughnut-shaped organ that sits at the base of every man's bladder. It produces a component of male semen, the fluid responsible for carrying and keeping alive male sperm cells. If the prostate fails to function properly, a man may not only experience problems with sexual function but also have difficulty with urination. If left untreated, some prostate malfunctions can become life-threatening.

No man can afford to ignore his prostate. Indeed, awareness of this little organ has increased in recent years. Public figures like retired U.S. Senator Bob Dole and golf legend Arnold Palmer went public with their diagnoses and recoveries from prostate illnesses – and rock star Frank Zappa and actors Telly Savalas and Bill Bixby died in their prime from prostate cancer.

The bulk of America's "baby-boom" generation is reaching middle age, the prime time for prostate trouble. Benign prostate hypertrophy, a nonfatal but bothersome enlargement of the gland, will affect half of all men over 40 and three-quarters of men over 65.

Even more frightening is the possibility of prostate cancer, a slow-growing cancer that will strike one man in eight. It will kill 31,900 American men this year, the American Cancer Society says, even though diagnostic tests and treatments are widely available. Sixty percent of newly diagnosed prostate-cancer cases and about 80 percent of deaths are in men 70 years old or older.

The number of reported prostate cases increased about 105 percent between 1986 and 1993—perhaps because of increased awareness and sophisticated diagnostics. Currently, 29 percent of all new cancer cases in American men are still prostate-related. Prostate cancer is three times more likely to strike African-American men than whites, and this could be due in part to a protein called TIMP-1. Scientists have recently identified levels of this protein to be 20 times greater in the prostate tumors of black men as compared to those of white men. Prostate-cancer incidence rises with age, so most men with prostate cancer die of old age rather than the disease.

All medical diagnoses and treatments should come from a licensed medical doctor, but men concerned about prostate health can lessen their suffering and hasten their recovery by studying how diet, exercise, and lifestyle changes can positively affect them. Men from other cultures have for centuries found prostate relief and even cures for cancerous growths through methods that American doctors may not have heard of. Some of these are outlined in this book.

But, as always, common sense and professional guidance are recommended.

An Anatomy Lesson

When the prostate gland is healthy, it is a truly remarkable little organ. It not only produces seminal fluid but also acts as a "storehouse" for male sperm.

THE PROSTATE
What It Is and What It Does

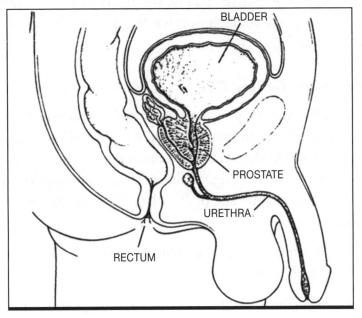

The prostate and the urinary tract share an outlet to the outside world, a tube known as the urethra—the reason that urine and semen come from the same opening at the end of the penis. Because this tube passes directly through the "doughnut hole" in the center of the prostate gland, enlargement of the gland can narrow the exit tube—thus causing the urinary problems familiar to so many men.

From *Prostate Problems,* by Charles E. Shapiro, M.D., and Kathleen Doheny, Dell Surgical Library.

Sperm are too tiny to see without a microscope. They are dark, tadpole-shaped cells that carry a man's genetic information. They are custom-designed to make the trip out of a man's body and into a woman's reproductive system and, if all goes according to biology, unite with a female ovum to create a new life.

Sperm cells are produced in a man's *testis* (see page 146), a small egg-shaped organ contained inside the scrotum, a bag of skin and sinew that hangs below the penis. After they are fully formed, sperm cells travel up the *vas deferens* to the prostate, where they are coated with a protective alkaline sheath. Without this chemical protection, sperm couldn't survive the acid environment of a woman's vagina.

The Hormones Do Their Part

At birth, the male prostate gland is only the size of a grain of barley. It doesn't begin growing until the onset of puberty, when *testosterone*, a sex-related chemical called a hormone, is produced in the nearby testes and signals the prostate to develop. The organ grows until about the age of 20, when the man reaches his full height.

Sexual arousal triggers a cellular exodus inside men with normal testosterone levels.

Sperm produced in the testes make a long journey upward, through yards of tiny tubes that lead to the prostate. Along the way they are supplied with high-energy milk sugar by the *seminal vesicles*, which then send the sperm for their alkaline coating of semen at the prostate gland. The finished product is sent through the ejaculatory duct and from there into the *urethra*.

When orgasm occurs, the prostate initiates a rhythmic series of contractions, or squeezes, around the urethra—a process known as ejaculation. The muscle contraction propels three or four bursts of semen outward at intervals of about one second.

FRONTAL VIEW OF
PROSTATE AND PUBIS

From *Prostate Problems,* by Charles E. Shapiro, M.D., and Kathleen Doheny. Dell Surgical Library.

When arousal is triggered but orgasm is delayed, an uncomfortable condition called *prostatic congestion*—or "blue balls"—can occur. Doctors don't agree on the risks of physical damage from this condition. But they do say relief is always close at hand—release of the semen through masturbation is the usual cure.

How Age Changes the Prostate

It is not unusual for a man's prostate to become larger as he grows older. By age 65, three out of four men suffer with some kind of prostate disorder. The presence of androgens—male hormones—makes the prostate grow, and these are chemicals most men wouldn't want to do without.

Simple changes in body chemistry create the prostate enlargement. The changing body uses hormones, medications, food, and other chemicals in new configurations, and organs sometimes receive "false messages" and react in ways that don't seem to make biological sense.

UPPER PART OF UROGENITAL SYSTEM
(DETAIL)

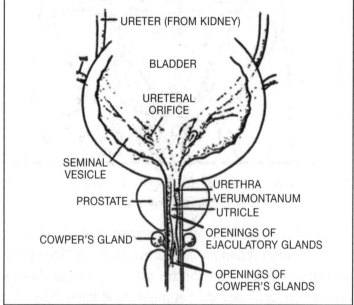

Statistics show that the average man's prostate begins growing at age 40 and begins to cause trouble of some kind by the time he reaches age 50. After that age, one in three men will require medical help for prostate problems. In most cases, the symptoms are not pronounced until the condition is well advanced.

Sometimes, the problem is easily solved. Urinary difficulty, one of the trademarks of prostate trouble, can also have other causes.

Men in their 60s and 70s sometimes find their urinary problems solved when they stop taking antihistamine medicine for colds or allergies. These drugs can cause contraction of the smooth muscle that surrounds the bladder neck and the prostate, which causes "urinary shutdown." Antihistamines don't seem to affect young men the same way. However, overindulgence in alcohol, especially beer, can cause acute urine retention in men of any age.

Prostatitis

The most simple-to-treat prostate problem is called *acute prostatitis*, or inflammation of the prostate. This bacterial condition affects old and young men alike and is easily spotted by a rapid onset of painful urination, pain at the base of the penis, and the presence of a cloudy fluid at the tip of the penis, as well as fever and chills.

Men with these symptoms should see a doctor immediately, as the symptoms can also indicate venereal disease. Treatment is a simple series of antibiotics.

Chronic prostatitis is a similar form of prostate inflammation that is more difficult to treat. There is seldom a bacterial cause for the condition, which creates a need to urinate frequently, a lessened desire for sex, and sometimes impotency—the inability to sustain an erection. The onset of chronic prostatitis is hard to pin down, because symptoms appear slowly and sometimes fade for months at a time.

The emotional toll of chronic prostatitis may be its most disturbing symptom. The sufferer may feel hopeless or depressed at his prospects for recovery, and his lack of sex drive may become a self-defeating resignation to permanent impotence.

Because of its sporadic nature, some doctors hesitate to treat chronic prostatitis with surgery or drugs. Many men find relief simply by talking about the problem with an understanding counselor, clergyman, or companion. Others find that a good exercise program brings welcome relief still others can get help through herbal cures and soothing baths, some of which are detailed later in this volume.

• CHAPTER 2 •

Benign Prostatic Hypertrophy

Benign Prostatic Hypertrophy (BPH):
Causes, Symptoms, Medical Treatments

Jim R., a 57-year-old personnel administrator, knows how many tiles there are along the baseboards in both his bathrooms. He'd counted them over and over while he waited to finish urinating.

He'd spent so much time in the john in the past few months he'd started to feel like a stranger in the rest of the house.

"I thought I'd broken a gasket there for a while," Jim said. "No sooner would I lie back down after going to the bathroom for the second time in the night than I'd feel like I had to go again. I couldn't make it through the second quarter of a ball game before I'd have to leave the room. It was getting embarrassing. And then it started to hurt."

Jim dislikes doctors and hospitals, but he swallowed his fear long enough to visit his family doctor.

After a physical that included a blood test and a digital rectal exam, Jim's doctor gave him the news.

"I just sat there and wondered, "What the heck is benign prostatic hypertrophy?" Jim said.

Benign prostatic hypertrophy, or BPH, affects half of all men over 50 and three-quarters of those over 65. The condition is entirely unrelated to cancer, but in its extreme forms it can be life-threatening.

BPH is an enlargement of the prostate from double its normal size up to grapefruit proportions. Experts aren't sure what causes the condition. Some say a drop in testosterone levels. Others say it is caused by changes in how the body metabolizes hormones. Genetics, scarred-over injuries, and various surgical procedures—including vasectomy—have been linked to an increased incidence of prostate enlargement. Some types of sexual activity can cause the prostate to swell. Whatever its exact cause, the primary diagnosis is usually hormonal imbalance.

COMPARISON OF NORMAL AND SWOLLEN PROSTATES

Normal Prostate   Enlarged Prostate

From *Prostate Problems,* by Charles E. Shapiro, M.D., and Kathleen Doheny, Dell Surgical Library.

Prostatic hypertrophy is practically undetectable until its later stages, because it develops slowly over many years. As the enlargement progresses, though, the man may experience pain in the groin or lower back, or he may feel a slight discomfort when he sits down.

As the condition progresses, sexual performance may be affected. Ejaculation can become painful, and a man may find himself ejaculating prematurely. He may even have intermittent bouts of impotence.

Some patients find that their headache remedy, ulcer or bowel medicine, or commonly used medications for depression or high blood-pressure are making their prostate disorders worse. A list of drugs that commonly complicate potency problems appears in Chapter 10.

Other men's prostates grow to a certain point and then stop. Enlargement doesn't necessarily mean the problem will become progressively worse. About 80 percent of men found to have mild BPH decide to delay treatment. Doctors call this option "watchful waiting"—going about your ordinary routine while keeping a careful watch for changes. Some men see their symptoms improve spontaneously, but not everyone is so lucky. For a man with a growing prostate, urination frequently becomes painful. Less urine is able to pass through the penis as the prostate slowly squeezes shut the urethra—the passageway between the bladder and penis. The prostate grows upward against the bladder, narrowing the duct that routes urine to the urethra. Sometimes, urination slows to a trickle. The bladder feels uncomfortably full. The man finds himself waking up frequently in the night to drain off whatever he can.

This situation can become life-threatening if it is allowed to continue unchecked and "strangle" the urinary tract.

In a worst-case scenario, the urine sits in a distended bladder, the chances of infection increasing as time passes. The bladder becomes inflamed, bladder stones may form, and the urine backs up into the kidneys. This leads to complete kidney shutdown, which can create fatal uremic poisoning of the bloodstream.

Fortunately, medical intervention is almost certain before these dire straits are reached. The vast majority of men die WITH a prostate problem, not FROM one. The key to preventing the pain of BPH is early detection and treatment.

SOME PROSTATE WARNING SIGNS:

- Pain in the prostate area
- Pain in the lower back
- Discomfort when sitting
- Painful urination
- A weak stream of urine
- A continual feeling of fullness in the bladder
- Waking several times at night to urinate, with only a small amount voided
- Painful ejaculation
- Intermittent impotency
- Dribbling

A Medical Diagnosis of BPH

Jim's initial doctor visit was just what he'd expected—a little unnerving. The questions were intense: "How often do you urinate, day and night?" "How steady is the flow?" "Do you have to stand and wait a while before the flow starts?"

"How often do you have sexual intercourse?" "Do you have pain on ejaculation?" But based on his answers, Jim's doctor ordered a full BPH evaluation.

His were only some of the methods doctors use to diagnose prostate troubles. Tests include the following:

DIGITAL RECTAL EXAMINATION

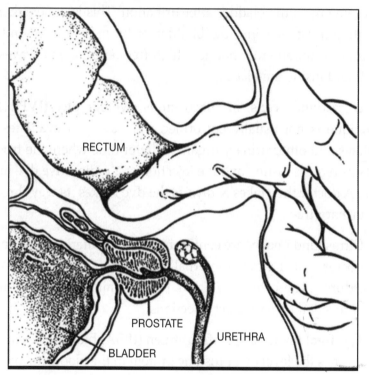

The doctor feels inside the rectum with a gloved finger. Because part of the prostate lies against the wall of the colon, doctors can detect abnormalities and tender spots with the touch of a finger.

Cystoscopy: A special viewing tube is inserted through the penis, which enables the doctor to view the obstruction and evaluate any damage the obstruction may have done inside the bladder. (A local anesthetic is used.)

Postvoidal and urine-flow measures: Sometimes doctors have a patient drink a large amount of fluid, to create a full bladder. The man then urinates into a funnel with a flow meter attached. This records the speed of the urine stream and the amount of urine produced. This test can determine if there is an obstruction in the urethra and can also provide an important "baseline" measure for later tests.

A postvoidal residual measure determines the amount of urine that remains in the bladder after urination. This is done either by inserting a catheter into the bladder or by using ultrasound, an imaging technique that bounces high-frequency sound waves off the liquid inside the bladder.

Ultrasound scans, or intravenous pyelography (IVP): This technique is not usually performed right away. It evaluates the kidneys and other urinary organs to determine where the trouble is. IVPs require fasting and the injection of a radioactive dye into a vein. A doctor then takes X-rays as the dye makes its way through the urinary tract.

Ultrasound images are configured on computer screens, giving the doctor a clear view of internal organs without use of invasive procedures. These tests rule out prostate ailments like tumors, prostatitis and urinary-tract infections.

The **Total prostate-specific antigen (tPSA) blood test**: This test determines the level of a prostatic protein in the bloodstream. This substance, produced by the prostate cells to keep seminal emissions liquid, is actually produced by normal as well as cancerous cells. However, cancerous cells produce an elevated quantity. When this level is read at 4 ng/ml, it is considered normal. A reading between the normal level and up to 10 could indicate the presence of prostate cancer. A reading above 10 is considered a strong indication of cancer.

A number of factors besides cancer can cause an elevated PSA, including benign prostatic hyperplasia, prostate infection, recent ejaculation, and even a digital rectal exam. In fact, as many as two out of three men who have biopsies due to elevated PSA levels are found not to have cancer. Several complimentary tests have been developed that your doctor may choose to use in addition to, or in replace of, the standard PSA test.

The **free PSA (fPSA) ratio test** measures the amount of PSA that is floating freely in the blood. Researchers found that men with cancer often have lower levels of free PSA than do those men whose PSA is elevated for other reasons, such as BPH. The fPSA test is often used in patients who have already had a total PSA test that showed elevated PSA levels. The fPSA test is more sensitive than the PSA test in diagnosing borderline cases and can help the physician and patient make a choice between surgery or another type of therapy. If the level of free PSA is below 25 percent, it is considered a strong indicator of prostate cancer and a biopsy is recommended.

Your PSA level can be evaluated by comparing it to the levels of other men in your same age group by performing an **age-specific PSA evaluation.** Because the PSA level *naturally rises with age* your doctor may decide to look at your PSA levels in relation to those of other men in your age group. This test, however, is not considered accurate alone and is often used in conjunction with other tests to get a more complete picture.

The **PSA velocity test**: Doctors use this test to track your PSA levels over a period of time. A steady rise in a man's PSA level can indicate the presence of cancer. In order to get an accurate reading, your doctor will follow your PSA levels by taking blood tests three times a year for two years. This allows him to compare the earliest results with later ones to determine the potential for cancer being present.

A protein called PSTF-1 is found in the urine of men with prostate cancer. The new noninvasive **PSTF-1 urine test** screens specimens for this protein to determine if a prostate is cancerous. Since it has a 90 percent accuracy rate in identifying prostate cancer, some researchers are calling it the new "gold standard" in prostate-cancer diagnosis.

Medical Treatments for BPH

Millions of dollars and hours have been poured into research on BPH—its causes and cures. Research has found three major options for men whose symptoms are intolerable and whose medical workups indicate a BPH-related blockage of the urinary tract.

These are medications, surgery, and "investigational methods," treatments that are still under study but are currently performed by qualified doctors.

Medications are usually the first step in dealing with a surly prostate.

Alpha-blockers: Hawk-eyed doctors in Wisconsin in 1991 found a link between blood-pressure medication and relief from BPH symptoms. Terazosin (brand name: "Hytrin") is usually prescribed for high blood pressure. It works by dilating, or widening, the blood vessels. A 1991 study at the Medical College of Wisconsin found the drug also relaxed the muscles at the neck of the bladder, bringing relief of blocked urine flow to 59 percent of BPH-affected men on a large (10 mg) dosage. Prazosin (brand name: Minipress) and doxasozin (brand name: Cardura) had similar effects on BPH patients.

The downside of alpha-blockers is their many side effects, which include sharp drops in blood pressure, dizziness, tiredness, and impotence. Not everyone can take these drugs.

Another class of medications now growing in popularity is called the *luteinizing hormone-releasing hormone (LH-RH) agonists.* They include *leuprolide* (brand name: Lupron) and *nafarelin acetate* (brand name: Synarel). They work by blocking production of testosterone, the male hormone that signals the prostate to grow. They are usually used to treat prostate cancer. The medicine is injected once a month and shrinks the prostate gland by cutting off testosterone.

LH-RH agonists almost always produce impotence. Other side effects include headaches and hot flashes.

Flutamide (brand name: Eulexin) also shrinks the prostate through hormone manipulation, but its side effects include stomach upset and breast development.

In 1992, the FDA approved the drug *Finesteride* (brand name: Proscar), a prostate shrinker discovered through a group of Caribbean natives a researcher found in the Dominican Republic.

In the mid 1970s, the scientist told his colleagues about the ethnic group, no member of which ever developed BPH or male-pattern baldness. Closer examination of the group found a genetic trait that created a deficiency of a blood protein called 5-alpha reductase. This protein usually interacts with testosterone to signal prostate growth. Without it, the natives' prostates remained small throughout adulthood.

Over several years, chemists at Merck Pharmaceuticals Co. developed *Finesteride,* (marketed as Proscar), a chemical that blocks production of 5-alpha reductase. Clinical trials have shown that about a third of the men who take the drug experience improved urine flow and marked prostatic shrinkage.

Disadvantages include a long waiting period before results are seen, occasional impotence, and an indefinite effectiveness—one study found that four months after discontinuing the drug, prostate symptoms had returned to their pre-treatment conditions. It simply doesn't work for two-thirds of the men who try it.

Another drawback to *Finesteride* is its effect on blood chemistry. Researchers say it lowers levels of other prostate proteins that are important to cancer diagnoses.

Finesteride can also affect women. Women of childbearing age, pregnant women, and those who may someday bear children are warned against handling the tablets, as the chemical can pass into the system through skin contact and cause abnormal sexual development in male fetuses.

Men who use *Finesteride* are warned to use condoms if they have intercourse with a fertile partner, as their semen can have a similar effect. Male children conceived by *Finesteride* patients may be born with malformed sex organs.

Researchers have experimented with combining *Finesteride* and alpha-blockers in the hopes that there would be an even greater improvement in prostate symptoms. However, the results were disappointing—with little to no improvement shown when used in combination.

Sometimes, medicine doesn't do the job or the symptoms are too advanced for pharmaceutical treatment. At this point, most medical doctors recommend prostate surgery.

Surgery

Dr. Charles Shapiro and Kathleen Doheny give detailed descriptions of surgical prostate treatments in their 1993 book *The Well Informed Patient's Guide to Prostate Problems*. Available options are simply outlined here:

Prostate surgeries used today include *open prostatectomy, transurethral resection (TURP), transuretheral microwave thermotherapy (TUMT), transuretheral needle abulation (TUNA), water-induced thermotherapy (WIT), transurethral incision (TUIP), balloon dilation,* and *laser surgery.*

TRANSURETHRAL RESECTION (TURP)
Removes Overgrown Prostate Tissue

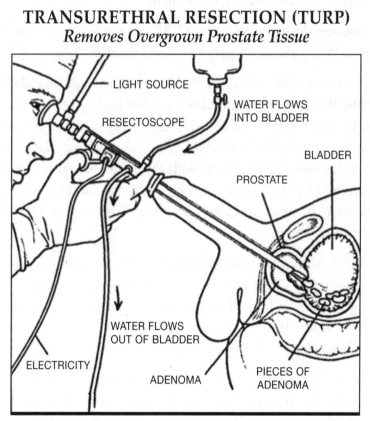

TURP consists of inserting an instrument through the penis and cutting away the overgrown prostate tissue. There is no skin incision. The operation takes 30 minutes to two hours and usually requires a general or spinal anesthetic. Samples of the excised tissue are then analyzed for cancer growth.

From *Prostate Problems,* by Charles E. Shapiro, M.D., and Kathleen Doheny, Dell Surgical Library.

Open prostatectomy is the most radical surgical procedure and is usually reserved for very large prostates or cancerous glands. Usually using general anesthesia, a doctor removes the offending tissue through an incision in the man's lower abdomen. Prostatectomy patients can expect a hospital stay of up to a week. About 85 percent of prostatectomy patients are left impotent, and 27 percent are left partially incontinent.

Transurethral resection, or **TURP,** is referred to as "the gold standard" in prostate surgery in several medical texts.

A curious side effect of TURP is "retrograde ejaculation." Because the incision traumatizes the tubes that carry semen to the urethra, most mens' bodies will, after surgery, send the semen backward into the bladder instead of out the usual exit. The ejaculate is then harmlessly eliminated with the urine. Sexual sensation is not affected by the surgery or retrograde ejaculation, doctors say, even though some couples find these "dry orgasms" a little disconcerting.

TUIP, or *transurethral incision,* uses the same instrument and anesthesia as a TURP. It is usually used on smaller prostates and younger men and involves no incision or removal of tissue. Patients report less retrograde ejaculation with this operation— only about 25 percent are affected.

In the last several years, new, less-invasive surgical treatments called thermal therapies have moved into the mainstream. These various therapies involve the heating of the prostate by several different methods. This heating often results in an improved urinary flow for the patient.

TUMT, or *transuretheral microwave thermotherapy,* is a fairly new outpatient treatment that is gaining popularity. During this treatment, a probe to monitor temperature is placed into the rectum.

A catheter containing a small microwave antenna is then placed into the urethra so that it lies close to the enlarged gland. The actual antenna extends into the prostate material, and cooling liquid is circulated through the tubing to protect the surrounding urethral tissue from excessive heating. The catheter is attached to an instrument that allows the doctor to direct microwave energy into the prostate. The high temperatures, created by the microwaves, heat and destroy the diseased tissue while the surrounding healthy tissues are left unharmed.

The treatment usually takes about one hour to complete. Despite no need for hospitalization, the TUMT patient can expect to have a urinary catheter for several days following the procedure due to the initial moderate to severe swelling of the prostate. Additionally, there is a risk of urinary-tract infections during the catherization period. The improvement in urinary flow follows the procedure by several weeks. After one or two years, the positive effects wear off in about half the men treated with TUMT and a repeat treatment is needed.

Also important to note is that the FDA released a public-health notification in October of 2000 regarding microwave thermotherapy for BPH in which it states its concern about some "unexpected procedure-related complications that have occurred since the marketing of these devices." According to the release, a number of factors could have contributed to these troubling injuries including oversedation of patients, who are then unable to communicate pain due to incorrect placement of the devices.

In the **TUNA,** or *transuretheral needle abulation* procedure, the doctor uses precisely controlled radio frequencies to heat the prostate. As in the TUMT procedure, a temperature probe is placed in the patient's rectum. A rigid catheter with an on-board telescope is then inserted through the urethra, which allows the urologist to easily see the prostate. Two needles, which actually serve as an antenna for the radio-frequency device, are inserted through the catheter into a swollen area of the prostate. The radio frequencies are then directed into the prostate. The needles are removed and reinserted into other swollen areas of the prostate.

The total outpatient procedure often lasts less than an hour. As with the TUMT procedure, the patient will have a urinary catheter for several days and the improvements will follow the treatment by several weeks. Since the TUNA treatment requires the repositioning of the catheter and needles several times during the treatment, some patients experience more discomfort and some bleeding. Heavier sedation may be needed to reduce discomfort. As with TUMT, about half of the men treated with TUNA will have a relapse of symptoms within a year or two and need an additional treatment.

Water-induced thermotherapy, or **WIT,** is a very new addition to the thermal-therapy family of treatments. In the WIT procedure, water is heated to 60 degrees Celsius and circulated through an insulated catheter placed in the man's urethra. At the end of the catheter is a balloon that allows the hot water to transfer heat directly to the prostate. The insulated catheter and precise water temperatures eliminate a need for the uncomfortable rectal-temperature probe used in other thermal therapies. Only a topical anesthetic is needed during the 45-minute procedure, and men report only mild discomfort. A urinary catheter is inserted after the procedure and kept in place for several days. Although the procedure has very few reported side effects and is considered relatively safe, a troubling 12 percent of patients need the urinary catheter for over a month following the procedure.

One of the latest treatments for BPH is the use of lasers on the obstructing tissues. This high-tech approach allows the surgeon to use intense light beams to accurately cut, coagulate, or vaporize tissues, with little or no bleeding.

Non-contact endoscopis laser ablation of the prostate (ELAP) is the most widely used laser method to date. In ELAP the surgeon directs the laser beam onto the prostate. The laser penetrates about 8 to 10 millimeters into the tissue, and the treated tissue coagulates—eventually creating a cavity.

In *Interstitial laser coagulation* (ILC), the laser is actually inserted into the prostate tissue. It is used to coagulate 5 to 10 different zones of tissue, which are then reabsorbed—reducing the overall size of the prostate.

A sapphire contact tip is used in *contact vaporization of the prostate*. This special coating causes the energy from the laser to be concentrated on the tip and allows the prostate tissues to be vaporized

LASER SURGERY OF
THE ENLARGED PROSTATE

From *Prostate Problems,* by Charles E. Shapiro, M.D., and Kathleen Doheny, Dell Surgical Library.

quickly and with less penetration. The surgeon draws the tip across the prostate, creating a cavity that relieves the swelling.

Holium laser resection of the prostate allows the surgeon to make a number of bloodless cuts in the prostate and remove pieces of prostate tissue. The advantage to this technique is that actual prostatic tissue can be removed and checked for cancer.

Doctors report less bleeding and quicker postoperative recovery time with laser surgeries. But these high-tech and still experimental procedures are often too expensive for many patients, and their long-term effectiveness isn't determined.

There are medical drawbacks to these less-invasive and quicker surgeries. Because no tissue is removed from the prostate, doctors can't test for cancer cells. And the long-term benefits of transurethral incisions are questioned, since many patients must return for more surgery when their prostates again enlarge and block urinary flow.

Balloon dilation of the prostate is another popular treatment, and is especially useful for prostate sufferers whose other health problems make more invasive surgery risky. Using an instrument similar to the TURP, a doctor inserts the tip of a carefully measured balloon into the prostate through the urethra. As the balloon inflates, it spreads open the prostate, widening the passage to the bladder by splitting the interfering prostate tissue.

Studies show that balloon dilation brings long-term relief to up to 60 percent of patients, but many must return for retreatment. Also, no prostate tissue is removed for routine cancer analysis. The procedure is sometimes done on an outpatient basis.

As with any surgical procedure, there are certain risks of bleeding, anesthesia reactions, infection, scarring and postoperative

BALLOON DILATION OF THE PROSTATE

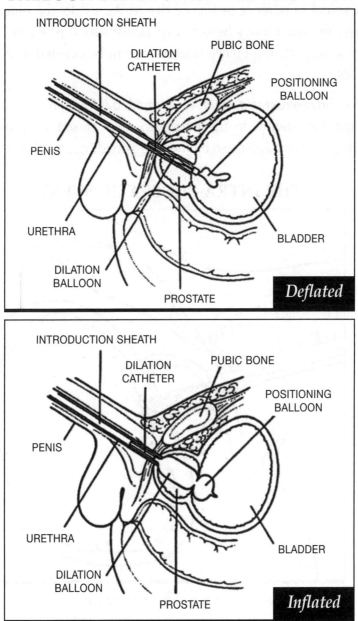

From *Prostate Problems,* by Charles E. Shapiro, M.D., and Kathleen Doheny, Dell Surgical Library.

incontinence. Ten percent to 15 percent of men report problems with sexual impotence or loss of desire. As a rule, the older the patient, the more likely he is to experience sexual problems after prostate surgery. Impotence treatments will be covered in a later chapter.

An *intra-prostatic stent* is a small device that is inserted through the urethra to the narrowed area caused by prostatic swelling. The braided-mesh biomedical-wire device is released and

THE INTRA-PROSTATIC STENT

The stent pushes back the prostate, opens the urethra and relieves urinary problems.

From *Prostate Problems,* by Charles E. Shapiro, M.D., and Kathleen Doheny, Dell Surgical Library.

opens like a spring, pushing the swollen tissues back and widening the urethra. Complications from this device include reports of irritation, debris forming on the stent, and a higher incidence of urinary-tract infections.

Doctors and researchers don't rely solely on chemicals and surgeries for treatment. They constantly search for new solutions to this age-old problem.

Because medicine is rapidly developing, the procedures outlined here may have been developed while the book went to press. Those interested in the latest studies on BPH treatments may contact the urology department of their community teaching hospital or university medical center.

• C H A P T E R 3 •

Nature's Way of Dealing With Enlarged Prostates

We Americans are fascinated by medical science and high technology. We hold our doctors in awe and take their word as gospel truth—sometimes to our own detriment. We look to them for quick solutions to health problems we develop through years of bodily neglect or abuse.

Most thinking people know there are other solutions to medical problems, sources of relief that lie far from the antiseptic atmosphere of the pharmacy or operating theater. Relief, and sometimes a cure, can be found in nature. This statement can be safely made without casting doubt on the expertise of the doctors who study prostate and urinary-tract functions.

Many healthy men say their lack of prostate problems is due to good common sense—eating right, exercising, and taking the right balance of vitamin and minerals. But to the man accustomed to high-fat meals and a low-energy lifestyle, surgery may seem an easier alternative than a lifestyle change... until his doctor schedules a prostate procedure for him!

We all know that a good diet can provide your body with the

vitality needed for a healthy, active life. Perhaps the role of diet is best illustrated by that raspy-voiced, muscle-bound cartoon sailor man named Popeye.

Popeye's superhuman feats and hair's breadth rescues are fueled by spinach—the lowly leafy-green vegetable he forever carries, canned, in his bosom or back pocket. After tearing open the tin and swallowing down its contents, Popeye's strength bursts forth in a frenzy of bulging biceps and karate kicks.

Popeye illustrates an old saw: "You are what you eat." Diet can, indeed, provide us with seemingly unlimited strength and energy. The only thing wrong with Popeye's spinach is the can. He really should eat the spinach fresh.

But what does a good diet have to do with the prostate gland?

Health comes from the inside out. No one can appear outwardly healthy if he isn't putting healthy things inside. A proper diet provides the right nutrients for every organ of the body—including the prostate.

Processed and refined foods contain chemical flavor enhancers and preservatives that are carefully controlled by the Food and Drug Administration—because in large doses or under certain storage conditions, these chemicals are poisonous to humans. It's no surprise that study after study finds that cutting out processed foods and increasing our intake of natural and fresh food brings about better health—including a healthier prostate.

Researchers are studying several natural substances that are known to shrink the prostate—and even cure cases of benign prostatic hypertrophy.

Zinc

For more than 50 years, science has known that seminal fluid from a healthy prostate contains a high concentration of zinc. One ejaculation may contain nearly all the zinc absorbed by the body in one day.

Zinc deficiency in males can have serious consequences. It can lead to infertility and, in severe cases, impotency. Some evidence also shows that a lack of zinc may be the culprit in cases of chronic prostatitis.

In a study at Chicago's Cook County Hospital, the zinc content of semen samples from chronic prostatitis patients was measured against samples taken from normal, healthy men. The prostatitis sufferers' semen contained 50 milligrams of zinc per milliliter. The normal samples contained an average of 448 milligams per milliliter—more than nine times that of the prostatitis sufferers.

In another study, 200 male patients with prostatitis were given zinc supplements. With doses of 11 to 34 milligrams a day over four months, more than 70 percent of the men reported that their symptoms disappeared.

In St. Louis, a Washington University School of Medicine study indicated that zinc has antibacterial properties that may protect the prostate from infections. However, men already infected with bacterial prostatitis did not respond to zinc therapy.

The U.S. governments recommended daily allowance (RDA) of zinc is 15 milligrams a day for adults. Although some nutritionists disagree, many doctors say it is difficult to get enough zinc from a normal diet. In fact, one study (funded by the National Cancer Institute) found that men who were taking a supplement of zinc daily decreased their risk of prostate cancer by 45 percent.

Shellfish are the best dietary source of zinc. Oysters contain between 70 and 100 grams of zinc apiece—and their reputation as an aphrodisiac is legendary!

As a daily supplement, men should take no more than 30 milligrams of zinc each day. Not all zinc taken into the body is absorbed, and too much may interfere with the body's processing of minerals like iron and copper.

Other sources of zinc include eggs, cheese, legumes, seeds, nuts, peas, corn, carrots, brown rice, garlic, onions, wheat germ, whole grains, and brewer's yeast; however, eggs and cheese should be eaten in moderation. Their fat and cholesterol contents have been linked to heart disease.

Selenium

Some researchers say selenium—another trace element the body needs in tiny amounts—is a good preventive medicine for prostate sufferers. It improves your blood's ability to deliver oxygen, keeps your tissues elastic and firm, and helps keep the retinas in your eyes healthy. There have also been reports of the mineral reducing anxiety and causing an overall sense of well-being. Now, however, some convincing studies have shown a connection between selenium and a reduced risk of prostate cancer.

Selenium, a metal, is normally found in rocks and soil. The mineral is passed through soil into the foods we eat. In fact, studies have shown that just living in areas that have low levels in the soil can increase the risk of getting prostate cancer.

A landmark 10-year study, conducted by the University of Arizona, followed 1,312 people living in areas of the United States that have low levels of selenium in the soil. The study was originally intended to look at the mineral's effect on skin cancer.

The researchers were shocked when their work revealed that a daily selenium supplement could cut your overall risk of getting cancer by an incredible 50 percent. Men in the study, who were given 200 micrograms of selenium a day had a 63 percent reduction in their risk of prostate cancer as compared with those who received a placebo. The head researcher on the University of Arizona study, Dr. Larry Clark, speculated in a later interview that a particular protein found in the prostate is responsive to selenium and probably helps to protect the prostate against "oxidative damage." The selenium-treated group of the ground-breaking study also had 46 percent fewer lung cancers, 58 percent fewer colorectal cancers, and half as many deaths from cancer.

Researchers from the Harvard School of Health conducted a study comparing men's selenium levels and their risk of developing prostate cancer. As with the case with the earlier University of Arizona study, the Harvard researchers found that more selenium in your diet might reduce your risk of prostate cancer.

The current recommended daily allowance for grown men is 70 micrograms. However, typical recommendations may range from 70 to 200 micrograms a day. You can add more selenium to your diet by eating foods typically higher in the mineral, such as fish, poultry, meat, whole grains, Brazil nuts, and vegetables.

Too much selenium in the diet can have undesirable side effects, such as hair loss, teeth loss, and fatigue. It is generally recommended that you should not exceed 400 micrograms a day.

Essential Fatty Acids

Dr. W. Devrient, a German nutritionist whose work is well-known in Europe, believes that essential fatty acids are vital in healing and maintaining prostate tissue.

Research shows that men need five times the fatty acids women do, to help maintain the elasticity of cell tissue. Seeds, nuts, and the oil from flaxseed are all excellent sources of these important nutrients.

Devrient tells prostate patients to consume lots of seeds and nuts daily—especially pumpkin, squash, and sesame seeds. Almonds, too, are a good source of fatty acids. Pumpkin seeds and pumpkin-seed oil are Devrient's favorites. He calls them "an inexhaustible source of vigor offered by Mother Nature."

Rick R., one of Devrient's patients, testifies to the effectiveness of this humble healer. He developed prostate problems when only 40 years old. His doctor recommended surgery, but Rick's brother had undergone a similar operation two years before. He'd advised Rick to avoid the procedure at any cost.

Instead, Rick began pumpkin-seed therapy. He ate pumpkin seeds by the handful, about 20 or 30 pounds of seeds a year. It's been five years since the doctor ordered surgery, and Rick says he walks away from each checkup with a clean bill of health.

Flaxseed oil is an alternative for those who don't care for crunchy seeds and nuts, which are sometimes difficult for denture wearers to chew. *Unrefined, cold-pressed flaxseed oil*, only one table-spoon per day mixed with unsweetened yogurt or low-fat cottage cheese, is used throughout Europe in treatment of BPH. It is also used to treat *cancer, arteriosclerosis, arthritis,* and *eczema.*

As shown in the chart that follows, the body converts the *linoleic* and *linolenic acids* in the unrefined flaxseed oil into prostaglandins, chemicals that are present in healthy prostates, seminal fluids, lungs, kidneys, thymus glands, and brain tissues. Several prostaglandins act as vasodilators—opening up veins and capillaries and increasing blood flow.

THE PRESENCE OF POLYUNSATURATED FATTY ACIDS IN VARIOUS OILS
and Their Influence on Human Diseases

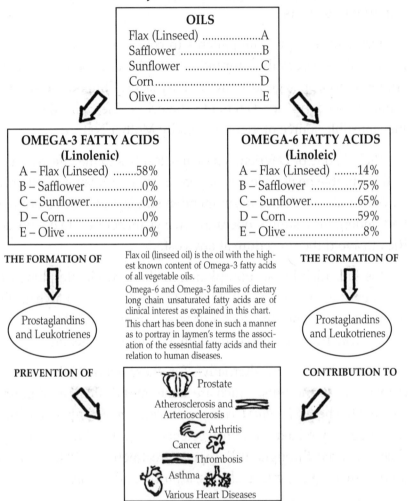

OILS

Flax (Linseed) ....A
Safflower ....B
Sunflower C
Corn.....................................D
Olive ....E

OMEGA-3 FATTY ACIDS (Linolenic)

A – Flax (Linseed) 58%
B – Safflower 0%
C – Sunflower..................0%
D – Corn 0%
E – Olive 0%

OMEGA-6 FATTY ACIDS (Linoleic)

A – Flax (Linseed) 14%
B – Safflower 75%
C – Sunflower................65%
D – Corn 59%
E – Olive 8%

THE FORMATION OF

Prostaglandins and Leukotrienes

PREVENTION OF

Flax oil (linseed oil) is the oil with the highest known content of Omega-3 fatty acids of all vegetable oils.

Omega-6 and Omega-3 families of dietary long chain unsaturated fatty acids are of clinical interest as explained in this chart.

This chart has been done in such a manner as to portray in laymen's terms the association of the essesntial fatty acids and their relation to human diseases.

THE FORMATION OF

Prostaglandins and Leukotrienes

CONTRIBUTION TO

Prostate
Atherosclerosis and Arteriosclerosis
Arthritis
Cancer
Thrombosis
Asthma
Various Heart Diseases

Flax oil (linseed oil) is the best seed oil for people with fatty degeneration, because the oil contains the largest amount of the most strongly dispersing essential fatty acid, the three-time unsaturated linolenic acid (LNA = linolenic acid = Omega-3).

LNA helps to disperse from our tissues deposits of the saturated fatty acids and cholesterol, which like to aggregate and which make platelets sticky. (Platelets play an important role in blood coagulation and blood-thrombus formation.) The oil has to be fresh and not exposed to light, oxygen, and heat, because these three agents destroy the essential fatty acids very rapidly. The oil should be unrefined, fresh, and not older than three months after pressing. (From *"The Complete Guide to Fats and Oils In Health and Nutrition"*.)

Los Angeles physician W.L. Cooper reported on an experimental *unrefined-flaxseed-oil* treatment administered to 19 prostate patients. Results included the following improvements:

- Increased sexual drive

- Increased energy

- A reduction in size of the prostate gland

- Increased urination

- Less residual urine

Note: There have been some recent reports suggesting an increased risk of prostate cancer with flaxseed-oil use. It is still yet unclear what form of flaxseed oil was used in those studies, and how the researchers attained their results. However, the benefits of raw, unrefined, cold-pressed, flaxseed oil, as is recommended throughout this book, have been proven in studies across the world. We recommend you speak with your physician to determine your specific risks and benefits before adding any supplements to your diet.

ESSENTIAL-FATTY-ACIDS CONTENT OF COMMON VEGETABLE OILS

Source	Fat Content Total %	Essential Fatty Acids Linolenic	Linoleic	Both Essentials Total %
Linseed [1]	35	58	14	72
Soybean	18	9	50	59
Pumpkin	47	15	42	57
Walnut	60	5	51	56
Rapeseed [2]	30	7	30	37
Safflower	59	0	75	-
Sunflower	47	0	65	-
Grape	Trace	0	71	-
Corn	4	0	59	-
Wheat Germ	10	0	35	-

CONTINUED ON NEXT PAGE

Essential-fatty-acids Content of Common Vegetable Oils; *continued*

Source	Fat Content Total %	Essential Fatty Acids Linolenic	Linoleic	Both Essentials Total %
Sesame	49	0	54	-
Rice Bran	10	0	35	-
Cotton [3]	Trace	0	50	-
Peanut [4]	47	0	29	–
Almond	54	0	17	-
Macadamia	71	0	10	-
Cashew	41	0	6	-
Olive	20	0	8	-
Coconut	35	0	3	-
Palm Kernel	35	0	3	–

[1] Linseed (flaxseed) unrefined, cold-pressed
[2] Rapeseed (canola) contains toxic *erucic acid*
[3] Cottonseed contains common toxins
[4] Peanuts (damp) harbor a toxic fungus
Hemp (not listed above because it is illegal in the U.S.) provides both essential fatty acids)

Bee Pollen

Many men who successfully treated their prostate symptoms with iron also swear by a supplement that seems to work well with zinc. *Bee pollen*—a natural substance created by honey bees to nourish their young—contains every nutrient known by doctors to maintain good health. Its positive effect on prostatitis is remarkable.

Nutritionists say bee pollen contains more than 5,000 enzymes and coenzymes—far more than any other food. Enzymes are essential to healing and digestion and are said to protect against premature aging. It is also packed with important vitamins, proteins, and nucleic acids—some authorities call it "nature's perfect food."

HIGH DESERT HONEYBEE POLLENS™
CHEMICAL ANALYSIS

PROTEIN	
7.1 GRAMS PER OZ (RDA 12 GRAMS)	

Standard chemical analysis identifies only 18 of the 22 amino acids present in pollen.

AMINO ACIDS	MGs PER OZ
Cystine	36.855
Lysine	366.360
Histidine	138.590
Arginine	292.520
Aspartic	542.440
Threonine	236.856
Serine	289.680
Glutamic	585.040
Proline	505.520
Glycine	267.520
Alanine	309.560
Valine	280.592
Methionine	94.004
Isoleucine	230.040
Leucine	377.720
Tyrosine	139.440
Phenylalanine	236.850
Tryptophan	49.700

Note: *Realities of Nutrition* states a person using the RDA to choose protein foods might not get enough of all essential amino acids. Bee pollen contains all essential amino acids.

MINERALS	MGs PER OZ
Calcium	42.383
Iron	2.118
Potassium	158.675
Phosphorus	121.706
Sodium	2.693
Iodine (in MCGs)	6.237
Magnesium	27.675
Zinc	1.460
Copper	.221
Boron	.604
Barium	.136
Chromium(less than)	.010
Manganese	1.395
Strontium	.094

MISCELLANEOUS	GRAM PER OZ
Carbohydrates	5.15
Fiber	1.02
Reducing Sugars	8.25
Ash	.65
CALORIES PER OUNCE	.90

VITAMINS	MGs PER OZ
A – 232,470 I.U.*	
Alpha Carotene	.031
Beta Carotene	.122
B1 (Thiamine)	.198
B2 (Riboflavin)	.459
B3 (Niacin)	2.551
Bˆ (Pyridoxine)	.119
B12 (Cyanocobalamin)	.00002
Biotin	.002
Folic Acid	.201
Pantothenic Acid	.198
C – (Ascorbic Acid)	1.304
D – 9 I.U.*	
E – 2.194 I.U.*	

* International Units

RUTIN – Abundant. (Not measured in analysis) Of great importance for capillary strength.

ENZYMES – Active enzymes are needed to digest and assimilate nutrients. Chemical analysis measures only three of the many present in bee pollen.

ENZYME	UNITS PER GRAM
Amylase (USP Units)	2.550
(Needed to break down starch)	
Protease (USP Units)	64.400
(Needed to split proteins)	
Lipase (mm Units)	.085
(Needed to emulsify fats)	

FATTY ACIDS   2.807 GRAM PER OZ

Essential fatty acids, with carbohydrates and sugars, supply our energy requirements.

CHOLESTEROL   0 PERCENT

Bee pollen contains a higher content (11) of the healthful unsaturated fatty acids as opposed to saturated (9).

NOTE: Bee pollen also contains elements science is not yet able to isolate and identify. Some authorities believe it is precisely these elements often called the "magic" of the bee, which make bee pollen so effective.

NOTE: This important chemical analysis was conducted by an Independent testing laboratory on the justly famous enzyme-active High-Desert® PollenS™ blend. It does not apply to any other brand of bee pollen in the world. It you see this analysis, or any portion thereof, reprinted elsewhere you may be certain proprietary material is being used both incorrectly and illegally to persuade you another product has the same documented high nutrient count as blended High-Desert®. Source: C.C. Pollen Company, Arizona.

Dr. Bernard C. Jensen, one of America's foremost natural nutritionists, said in his book *Nature Has a Remedy* that "much has been said about pollen's helping glands in the body. All experiments on animals show it prolongs life—and helps to keep the glands in good order."

Researchers at the Nagasaki University School of Medicine in Japan and the University of Lund in Sweden did independent studies of *bee pollen* and prostate problems. Both reported marked reduction in prostatic swelling and inflammation, even in severe cases of *prostatitis*. Neither study reported any adverse side effects.

Of the 172 men with prostate disease in a Swedish-German study in 1988, all who were treated with oral doses of *bee pollen* reported a cessation of symptoms.

Bee-pollen therapy began about 40 years ago in Sweden, where beekeepers discovered how much better they felt after indulging in the natural tonic.

Dr. Erik Ask-Upmark, M.D., a professor at the University of Upsala, learned of the substance from a beekeeping patient in 1957. The patient had intermittent bouts of *prostatitis*, accompanied by severe localized symptoms and high fever. He'd found no relief from doctors—and Dr. Ask-Upmark could offer no solutions.

The patient decided to take *bee pollen* as a general tonic, to build up his strength for scheduled prostate surgery. Very shortly after he started taking the *bee-pollen* doses, the man noticed that his prostatitis was gone.

He continued taking the pollen, and his symptoms only returned once—after he'd stopped taking the pollen for two weeks. His urologist canceled the surgery.

Ludwik Frangor was 70 when he discovered the benefits of *bee pollen.* At that time, his heart was so diseased his doctor wouldn't let him mow the lawn. He had given up on sex—he was widowed, so his impotence no longer bothered him. As his condition deteriorated, his son suggested he move to a nursing home for 24-hour care. The suggestion changed his life—Ludwik decided he wasn't ready to die then.

"From then on, I made *honeybee pollen* the one unvarying and essential foundation of my rejuvenation program," he said. "This perfect live food has restored my manhood and brought me back to full vigor... I am never sick."

Frangor lived well into his 90s, even celebrating his 94th birthday in 1989 with a cross-country ski trip.

Studies at Yugoslavia's University of Sarajevo showed that bee-pollen therapy aids in cases of prostatitis and impotency—and may also cure some cases of male infertility. *Bee pollen* administered to a group of infertile men produced a measurable increase in sperm production. Scientists credited a gonadotropin hormone in the pollen with the gland stimulation.

Dr. James Van Fleet routinely treats BPH and *prostatitis* patients with *bee pollen.* He told of a patient named Bill G., whose *prostate gland* was so swollen he visited the rest room every 20 minutes. The problem was costing him much sleep and work productivity, and the pain in his lower abdomen and back was becoming unbearable.

Dr. Van Fleet gave Bill *bee pollen.* He recommended a dose of eight capsules a day, two with each meal and two at bedtime. In less than a month, Bill's most severe symptoms had eased, and within two months, he was sleeping through the night again.

Scientists in this country have tried without success to scientifically duplicate *bee pollen*. Its unique combination of vitamins, minerals, amino acids, hormones, carbohydrates, and fatty acids—all in just the right proportions—has left chemists flummoxed.

Natural nutritionists say that many kinds of *bee pollen* are available at natural-food markets, but savvy customers should look for granules or capsules made from *High Desert* sources. This type of pollen is made from many different types of plants indigenous to unspoiled areas of Montana and the Dakotas of the western United States. It is not damaged through heat-processing and is free of industrial pollution.

Larry R., 65, visited Dr. Van Fleet when his family doctor told him his prostate gland should be surgically removed. Van Fleet's tests revealed Larry had a zinc deficiency. The doctor prescribed his usual eight capsules of *bee pollen* but also had Larry take 10 milligrams of zinc with each meal.

Within 10 days, Larry noticed improvement. After a month, all signs of prostate problems had disappeared.

Dr. Norman Meyers ran into a stubborn problem with patient Ed J., 79. Although he took the same dosages of zinc and bee pollen as Larry R., his condition did not improve.

Essential fatty acids, in the form of *unrefined, cold-pressed flaxseed oil,* proved the missing element in Ed's diet. When he consumed a tablespoon of the oil in yogurt or low-fat cottage cheese each day, his symptoms responded immediately.

Drs. Van Fleet and Meyers say that even men whose prostates are healthy should follow their nutritional recommendations as a preventive measure. The table at the end of this chapter shows the amounts of supplements to take and when to take them. All are available from any reputable natural food store.

Prostatitis Cures: Helpful Herbs

John Heinermann, an anthropologist and herbalist from Utah, has several suggestions for men who suffer with prostatitis, either the bacterial type or the chronic one.

Heinermann says *goldenseal root* is especially helpful in reducing *prostatitis* symptoms. A recipe for goldenseal tea is included later in this volume—he recommends 3 half-cups every four hours. *Fluid goldenseal extract* is also available at natural-food stores; the dosage is 15 drops three times a day. Those who prefer capsules should take two every five hours.

Chaparral is another herb that helps a swollen prostate. Heinermann recommends 1 cup of *chaparral tea* twice daily, 10 drops of fluid extract three times a day or four capsules each day.

Yarrow and *mallow* are two anti-inflammatory herbs that some prostate sufferers swear by—they soothe pain and burning sensations. Users should drink 2 cups of tea per day or swallow four capsules of either herb daily.

Heinermann stresses the importance of easy exercise and a diet high in fatty acids, zinc, fruits, and vegetables. He also recommends the use of "liquid chlorophyll," a green make-it-yourself concoction that is packed with vitamins and minerals needed for a healthy body and prostate.

To make the mixture, simply puree Romaine-lettuce leaves, parsley, and celery in a blender, juicer, or food processor. Strain and drink a half-glass at a time. The juice is also available in premade form at health-food stores under the name "Kyo-Green."

PRESCRIPTION FOR A HEALTHY PROSTATE

Supplement	Breakfast	Lunch	Dinner	Bed
Bee-pollen capsules[1]	2	2	2	2
Zinc tablets	10 mg	10 mg	10 mg	-
Flaxseed oil[2]	One tablespoon at breakfast, mixed with low-fat cottage cheese, unsweetened yogurt, or tofu.			

[1] Or 1 to 3 tablespoons granulated bee pollen per day.

[2] Only unrefined, cold-pressed flaxseed oil is recommended.

• C H A P T E R 4 •

Flower Pollen and Royal Jelly: New Angles on Old Cures

Nature offers an abundance of relief for ailments of almost every part of the human body. Indeed, pharmacologists frequently find new medicines by examining folk remedies. *Digitalis*, a well-known treatment for heart-rhythm dysfunctions, comes from the common *foxglove*, a wild flower Native Americans used for healing for centuries. Bread mold, used by Dutch and German immigrants to bring down fevers and heal infected cuts, was later used to form *penicillin*—the first antibiotic "miracle drug."

Many Europeans swear by another such discovery made "in the back yard." *Flower-pollen extract*, a potent and proven help in cases of *prostate enlargement*, comes from eight species of wildflowers that grow in the Scania District of southern Sweden. This is not the same as the *bee pollen* discussed in Chapter 3: *Flower pollen* isn't taken in and digested by bees before being processed.

Cernitin, or *cernitex*, the major ingredient in flower pollen, increases body tissues' resistance to invasion by outside agents, thus creating an anti-inflammatory effect. The other pollens work to promote urination, which is typically suppressed by prostate disorders.

Although the word "pollen" might make one think of watering eyes and itchy noses, all allergens are processed out of the *flower pollen* before they are administered to patients. Double-blind tests performed by urologists at Upsala University in Sweden examined the effects of a substance on a group of BPH patients as compared with a similar group taking a harmless "placebo." They found the *flower pollen* extract to be authentically beneficial to 90 percent of the men who took it.

Long-term use of the substance has shown no ill effects. Even those whose prostates did not shrink under treatment reported drops in the intensity of their symptoms. An impressive 76 percent of those tested reported relief from dysuria, or difficult and painful urination, and 89 percent said their urine streams had increased markedly with the *flower-pollen* therapy.

These improvements are due to the extract's contracting effect on the smooth "detrusor" muscle, which is responsible for emptying the bladder.

Flower pollen also suppresses production of androgenic hormones in the prostate—the same hormones suppressed by *alpha-blocker* medications discussed in chapter 2. The *alpha-blockers,* however, suppress the hormones produced in the testes, and their use sometimes results in impotence and breast development. Because the *flower pollen* works specifically on the prostate, no such side effects have been reported by its users.

QUESTIONS AND ANSWERS
About Flower pollen extract Tablets and Their Therapeutic Effectiveness For Diseases of The Prostate Gland

Q. *What is flower-pollen-extract?*

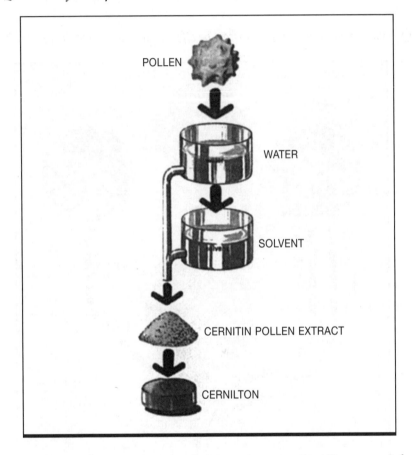

POLLEN

WATER

SOLVENT

CERNITIN POLLEN EXTRACT

CERNILTON

A. Flower-pollen extract is a therapeutic agent for diseases of the prostate the main ingredient of which is cernitin (or cernitex), a pollen extract from the pollen of eight plant species grown in the Scania District of South Sweden.

This substance has traditionally been used in Sweden for reinforcing physical strength as an anti-influenza agent, a nutrient, a tonic etc. Its effectiveness in treating prostatitis was discovered by Ask-

Upmark (Upsala University) in 1960 and was later confirmed in a double-blind test. Since its discovery, excellent results have been achieved in improving symptoms of chronic prostatitis and prostatic hypertrophy. Furthermore, since allergens are removed, it does not cause allergies and is a drug with extremely few side effects.

Q. *Why should flower-pollen extract be effective for diseases of the prostate?*

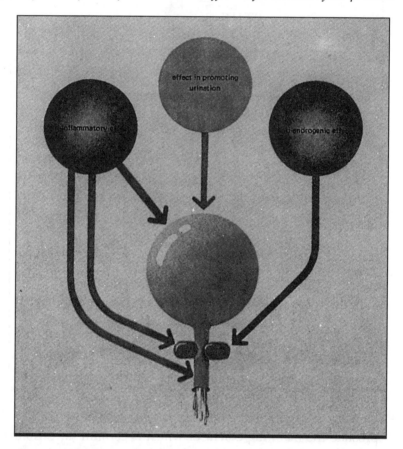

A. There is an effect in improving the various symptoms of diseases of the prostate due to its pharmacological action of promoting urination, its help in increasing levels of an important anti-androgenic hormone, and its effectiveness as an anti-inflammatory.

Q. *Why should flower-pollen extract be effective on dysuria due to diseases of the prostate?*

A. Measurements of urinary bladder pressure—electromyograms, for example—have clearly shown that the contractile power of the urinary bladder is increased in dysuria (due to mechanical pressure resulting from inflammation and hypertrophy of the prostate gland).

Q. *How does the effect of flower-pollen extract in promoting urination differ from that of other drugs?*

urination pressure

A. A study was made of its effect in promoting urination in animal experiments. The high value of 13.8 mmHg was shown in the group given flower-pollen extract orally for 14 days, as compared with 6.9 mmHg in the control group—and a higher urination pressure was shown than with other drugs supposed to produce the same effects.

Q. *What is meant by the anti-androgenic effect of flower-pollen extract?*

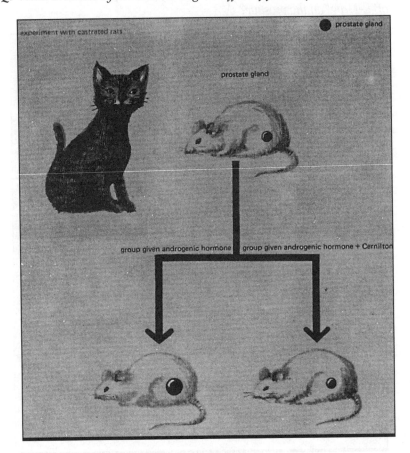

A. It has been confirmed that the prostate gland, and its hypertrophic portion in particular, is dependent on androgenic hormone and that flower-pollen extract acts specifically on the prostate gland, with antagonism to the androgenic hormone (Shida et al., Gunma University.)

Q. *What is the difference between the effect of flower pollen extract and that of"E-Drug"on the prostate?*

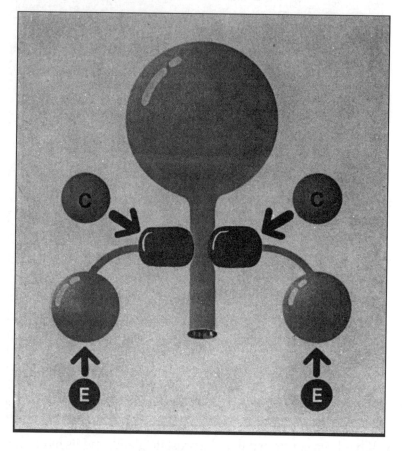

A. Both of these drugs have an anti-androgenic action, but it has been confirmed that flower pollen extract acts directly on the prostate gland whereas E-Drug depends on suppressing the secretion of androgenic hormone in the testicles.

Q. *Why does flower-pollen extract have an effect on chronic prostatitis?*

A. Flower-pollen extract increases the resistance of live tissue in the body and exerts an anti-inflammatory effect.

This is shown by its anti-inflammatory action against ovalbumin oedema in the filter-paper-pellet method and clinically is observed as disappearance of bacteria from the prostatic fluid and urine.

Q. *Are only older men suitable subjects for Flower Pollen Extract?*

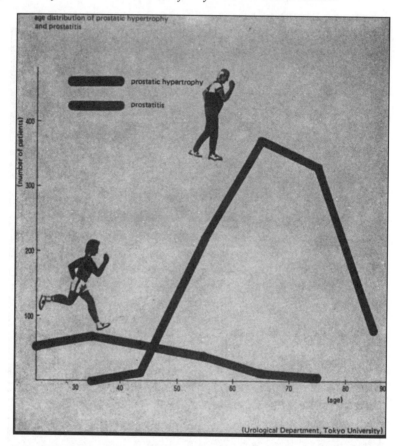

A. Chronic prostatitis is also observed in young people, and there have been more and more cases of prostatic hypertrophy from the late 40's onward. Therefore, Flower-pollen extract is indicated for dysuria due to diseases of the prostate in both young and old.

Q. *How does the prostate work?*

A. It is the glandular tissue that secretes the prostate fluid and accounts for 13 percent to 30 percent of the semen. It is thought to be important chiefly for the fusion of sperm and ovum.

Q. *What kind of Illness is prostatic hypertrophy?*

A. It is hyperplasia of benign tumor tissue that begins inside the gland in middle age in males (their 50s and 60s), gradually compresses the urethra, and causes difficulties in urination.

Q. *What is the clinical effect of flower-pollen extract on chronic prostatitis?*

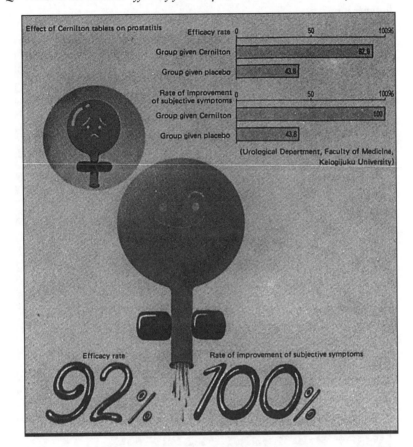

A. The effect on chronic prostatitis was studied by the double-blind method, using a placebo. The results obtained were for the overall assessment of flower-pollen extract: efficacy rate 92.9 percent, rate of improvement of subjective symptoms 100 percent. Excellent results.

Q. *What is the clinical effect of flower-pollen extract on prostatic hypertrophy?*

A. Viewing the effectiveness of flower-pollen extract on prostatic hypertrophy in the light of subjective and objective symptoms, such as dysuria, frequency of urination, residual urine, anuria, etc., in 65 patients in four institutions, researchers found that the extract improved all symptoms by about 80 percent.

Q. *What is the effect of flower-pollen extract on residual urine?*

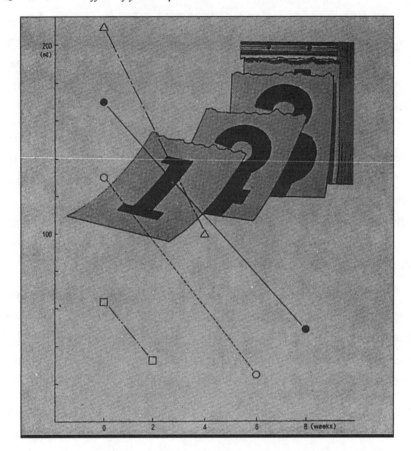

A. It is clear from the above diagram that this drug is also effective in reducing residual urine. Even when the amount of residual urine is large, success is achieved by prolonged administration.

Royal Jelly

Another natural product found to aid prostate sufferers is *royal jelly*, another gift of the honeybee. *Royal jelly* is manufactured in the hive for the sole consumption of the queen bee, whose life span sometimes surpasses five years. (Worker bees typically live only three to five weeks.)

Royal jelly is widely known as a dietary supplement, and medical research has confirmed its helpfulness in regulating blood pressure, enhancing the immune system, and easing arteriosclerosis and coronary deficiency. Rich in hormones, enzymes, vitamins, and amino acids like acetylcholine, *royal jelly* is thought to revitalize living cells. The first few doses sometimes produce a characteristic euphoria, which leads some to overexert themselves.

Two other components of *royal jelly* are *gamma globulin*—one of the body's natural antibiotics—and *proteic gelatin*, which builds up the collagen in connective tissues. Soviet scientists found that the jelly stimulates the nervous system and speeds glandular secretions, which may explain its reputation as an aphrodisiac.

Elena Groth, a naturopathic physician from Germany, has for years studied the effects of natural medicine on prostate complaints. The most remarkable cases include prostate-related sexual dysfunction—men who could not achieve an erection because of prostate symptoms. After a prescriptive dose of *royal jelly*, the majority of Groth's patients report a relief from burning urination and a return of potency in lovemaking.

The use of *royal jelly* in prostate cases was discussed at length at a convention of English and European urologists. Research continues into how and why this substance works, even on advanced cases of prostatitis and BPH.

Groth usually prescribes two royal jelly capsules three times a day, taken along with flower-pollen extract and a special seven-herb tea—a drink discussed in the following chapter.

Kombucha

Another alternative treatment from Europe is now available in North America. It is a tea-type drink, fermented from the *Kombucha* plant indigenous to Eastern Europe. It works by enhancing the body's metabolism and immune system, and is used throughout the Continent for kidney problems, liver problems, gallbladder problems, gout, migraine headaches, rheumatism, arthritis and more.

Dr. Rudolf Skienar, a German medical doctor, popularized the drink after he noticed the robust health of many elderly Eastern European and Russian peasants. The men boasted of their love-making prowess well into their 90s. Skienar found that all these peasants regularly drank *Kombucha* tonic, traditionally believed to have a magical ability to retard male aging.

Skienar prescribed 3 cups of *Kombucha* tea per day to a 48-year-old patient who saw it as his last resort before prostate surgery. After two weeks of the treatment, the patient reported increased urine flow and less burning when he urinated. After a month, the man regained his potency and was able to make love to his wife. All without surgery.

Kombucha has been found particularly effective in treating *impotency* in men with *prostate problems* and those whose sexual problem stems from high-blood-pressure medication.

Dozens of other plants have been found to have beneficial effects on men with *prostate problems*. Their functions and uses are detailed in the following chapter.

· CHAPTER 5 ·

Herbal Help for Prostates

We Americans usually turn up our noses at any cure not produced by high technology. We'll gladly swallow the foul-tasting, high-priced cough syrup prescribed by our doctors but wouldn't think of sipping tea made from an herb in the back yard, even if it was proven to eliminate coughs.

We have faith in modern medicine. We look to science for answers to life's questions. And while there is no doubt that science and technology have lengthened our lives and spared us countless diseases, we still tend to ignore or laugh at, nontechnological means of solving medical problems. Our open minds slam shut when talk of herbal cures comes up. Words like "poultice" and "elixir" conjure up visions of witch doctors, pipe-smoking grannies, or Wild West "snake-oil" peddlers.

As a society, we don't possess the rich history of natural remedies that is common to Europe. At one time, each village there had its herbalist—someone who knew what plants bring down childhood fevers and which tea helps bruises to heal.

Today, many Americans are more open-minded about herbal medicine. Prostate sufferers may also find relief in "nature's pharmacy." What follows is a listing of "prostate-friendly" herbs and compounds formulated from natural sources.

I am not, by any means, suggesting that herbs alone should be used to treat *prostatitis* or *prostatic hypertrophy*. I propose a marriage of modern and folk remedies. Herbs can be wonderful aids when used in conjunction with modern therapies.

The Small-flowered Willow Herb

The most potent herb for prostate troubles is an obscure one. So few herbalists wrote of it over the centuries it was almost "lost in time." It is the *small-flowered willow herb*, a water-loving plant that produces tiny white, pink, or rust-colored flowers.

Maria Treben, an Austrian herbalist, frequently prescribes a tea made from the herb to men whose prostate problems have laid them low.

"I beg you to show me a way back to health," a German gentleman wrote to Treben. "Give my family back their healthy father."

The man had suffered for years from *chronic prostatitis*. Medications prescribed by his doctor had left him with an ulcer and liver disorders, and still the man passed pus and blood in his stool. The man underwent prostate surgery with little effect. Additional medications and injections only worsened his condition. Finally, the man turned in despair to the herbalist.

Treben recommended he drink tea made from the *small-flowered willow herb*. Progress was slow at first, but within months his prostate inflammation was relieved. Even the liver disorder and ulcer cleared up.

Another man wrote to Treben to praise the lowly herb. While

he was hospitalized with a heart attack, the doctors found he also had a serious *prostate problem*. His medical condition ruled out an operation. The man read in a hospital pamphlet about the *small-flowered willow herb*, and decided he had nothing to lose in trying it.

"I began to drink 3 cups daily," he wrote. "After several days, I had no more complaints. I still drink 2 cups a day to ensure a complete recovery. I thank God from the bottom of my heart for the *small-flowered willow herb*. It is amazing that medicinal plants can give such results."

One case of the herb's effectiveness was termed a miracle by its beneficiary—a man who knows a miracle when he sees one.

Father Hohmann, a Catholic priest, was diagnosed with terminal prostate cancer. His doctor considered his case hopeless, and told the priest to make his peace and retire. But Father Hohmann wasn't ready to die. A local herbalist prescribed *small-flowered-willow-herb* tea. And, according to the clergyman, his cure was "nothing less than a miracle."

• INSTRUCTIONS •

SMALL-FLOWERED-WILLOW-HERB TEA

Preparation: Use only the fresh herb, and use the entire plant—stem, leaves and flowers. Mince them finely. Place a heaping teaspoon of the herb in 6 ounces of freshly boiled water. Cover and steep for three to four minutes; sip hot and unsweetened.

Frequency: 1 cup twice daily; one before breakfast and one in the evening at least 30 minutes before the final meal of the day.

■ *Damiana*

Herbalists also attest to the effects of *damiana,* an herb known as a stimulant to combat sexual weakness and as overall nerve tonic. In the earlier part of this century, American physician W.H. Myers used *damiana* extensively in his practice to treat impotency. "I find that in cases of partial impotence and other sexual debility, damiana's success is universal," he wrote. Dr. Steinmetz of Holland also attests to the effect of *damiana* and had excellent results with his patients.

• INSTRUCTIONS •

DAMIANA TEA

Preparation: Place 2 tablespoons of dried damiana in a cup. Add hot water and let steep for three to five minutes. Strain and drink hot.

Frequency: 1 cup daily.

Note: Do not overuse, as liver damage may result.

■ *Ginseng*

Probably the best-known of the so-called aphrodisiac herbs is *ginseng,* otherwise called "manroot." Available as a tea, extract, powder, liquid, capsule, or tablet, *ginseng* is credited with stimulation of androgen production, which assists in sex-gland functions. Magical and medicinal properties have been attached to this root for hundreds of years.

Dr. George Zofchak, an herbalist and a naturopath from central Pennsylvania, gives detailed advice on the uses of herbs in Mark Bricklin's *Practical Encyclopedia of Natural Healing.* He attests to the usefulness of *damiana* and has witnessed ginseng's powers as a general normalizing tonic for sexual function.

"*Ginseng* is not going to perform miracles...a cup of *ginseng tea* is not going to abolish a problem that stems from a deep psychological cause," Zofchak said, "but taken over a period of time, ginseng can have a general stimulating and normalizing effect, which may also help the sexual problem."

Zofchak recommends using *ginseng* grown in the United States, which is gathered from mountain areas where it grows wild. Other herbalists prefer Korean or Chinese-grown *ginseng*.

■ *Goldenseal*

A tea made from the herb *goldenseal* is an excellent aid for those with inflammation of the *prostate, colon,* and *rectum*—even if the taste is bitter and strong. It is useful, too, for treating *hair loss* and *athlete's foot* infections when a weak solution is applied to the affected area.

• INSTRUCTIONS •

GOLDENSEAL TEA

Preparation: Steep 1 teaspoon dried goldenseal root in 1 cup of boiling water for three minutes. Strain and sip hot. The tea may be sweetened with honey.

Frequency: several cups, taken throughout the day.

Note: Goldenseal should NOT be used by pregnant women.

■ *Mallow*

Mallow is an herb that provides nourishment to body tissues. It has a prestigious history dating back to Old Testament times. In

Job 30:4, the herb is mentioned as one of the few nourishments for people in times of famine.

Cold *mallow tea* could indeed help nourish an ill prostate. It is an excellent aid in cases of *bladder, stomach,* and *intestinal inflammation.*

• INSTRUCTIONS •

MALLOW TEA

Preparation: Soak 5 heaping teaspoons of the herb in 2 1/2 quarts of water overnight. In the morning, strain and warm slightly, but do not boil, before drinking.

Frequency: Drink 4 cups throughout the day.

Note: It is extremely important that mallow not be heated, as heat destroys its potent qualities.

Herbs That Aid in Urination

Several herbal formulas "specialize" in easing painful or difficult urination—a primary symptom of *prostatitis* or BPH. Try several to find the one that best suits your particular needs.

■ *Pygeum*

The bark of the African plum tree, Pygeum africanum, has long been a traditional African cure for prostate troubles as well as a variety of urinary-tract illnesses. Use of this healing bark has spread over Central and Eastern Europe and it is the No. one treatment for symptoms of BPH in France. The bark is believed to reduce testosterone levels, relax the muscles involved, and even increase secretions in the prostate gland.

Pygeum's ability to relieve many of the cumbersome symptoms of a swollen prostate has been proven in a number of studies. In fact, 65.5 percent of physicians and patients interviewed who have used Pygeum therapy rated the treatment as successful.

One landmark German study examined the effects of a 50 milligram Pygeum extract taken twice a day vs. a placebo. The Pygeum group had a 12 percent increase in urine volume compared with only 3.2 percent in the placebo group. Residual urine volume decreased an astounding 24.5 percent in the treated group, while the placebo group decreased 3.5 percent. Those in the Pygeum group also had measurable reductions in both their daytime and nighttime urination.

Judging by the results of a number of clinical studies, the recommended daily dosage of the pygeum is 100 to 200 milligrams a day divided into two doses. The brand most common in Europe and often used in clinical studies is manufactured by Rossa-Pharma and is known by the brand name Tadenan. Unfortunately, this product is not yet available on U.S. shelves. You can, however, find it through a number of Internet sources, including www.naturesdistributors.com and www.vitacost.com. Make sure to use the bark extract and not the dried bark, which has not been tested in any known studies.

■ *Saw Palmetto*

In five out of seven European studies, an extract from the saw palmetto berry came out a winner against BPH. Researchers found men taking saw palmetto extract had a reduced urgency to urinate and a greater urine flow. In fact, studies now show that saw palmetto appears to work as well as the standard BPH drug Finasteride in improving urinary symptoms with far fewer side effects.

One study of 305 patients found that a full 85 percent of the participants were reporting that the saw palmetto treatment effectively reduced their symptoms within three months. Significant improvements in symptoms were reported in another three-month study only 45 days into treatment with saw palmetto. Of the 505 men with mild to moderate symptoms followed in the three-month trial, 88 percent of them declared the therapy successful after 90 days. Researchers at the University of California recently concluded that saw palmetto is a safe and desirable treatment option for men who suffer from BPH.

There are a number of saw palmetto teas on the market; however, these preparations have not been studied. Because these teas do not contain the fat-soluble components of the supplement, they are most likely not effective. It is recommended that you use a saw palmetto extract and not a tea.

■ *Club Moss*

This mossy deep-woods trailing plant can aid in easing *inflammation of the testes* as well as *difficult urination*.

• I N S T R U C T I O N S •

CLUB-MOSS TEA

Preparation: Pour 1 pint of boiling water over 1 level teaspoon club moss. Steep for five minutes and drain.

Frequency: Drink only 1 cup daily on an empty stomach— best if used a half-hour before breakfast.

■ *Horsetail*

The *horsetail herb* is fairly common, growing wild in fields and meadows. It has no leaves or branches. Its shape resembles a slender pine tree, but it seldom grows taller than 10 inches. Sipping a cup of *horsetail tea*—with a little honey, if you wish—may promote urination.

• INSTRUCTIONS •

HORSETAIL TEA

Preparation: Pour 6 ounces of freshly boiled water over 1 heaping teaspoon of horsetail. Cover and steep for four to five minutes. Strain and sip hot.

Frequency: Use 1 cup daily.

■ Wild Thyme

Wild thyme can grow just about anywhere and likes lots of sun and heat. Its blossoms are small and deep purple and are a well-known diuretic.

• INSTRUCTIONS •

WILD-THYME TEA

Preparation: Pour 6 ounces of freshly boiled water over 1 heaping teaspoon of wild thyme, either fresh or dried. Cover and steep for three or four minutes. Strain and sweeten with honey.

Frequency: Drink 1 cup daily.

■ Stinging Nettle

Don't be intimidated by the mention of *stinging nettles* in the same breath as your urinary equipment. As daunting as it sounds, this 10-inch plant provides soothing relief to *suppressed urination* and *inflamed urinary tracts*.

The plant has drooping heart-shaped leaves and is covered

with protective "stinging" hairs. If you pick it fresh, be sure to wear gloves.

• I N S T R U C T I O N S •

STINGING-NETTLE TEA

Preparation: Pour 6 ounces of freshly boiled water over 1 heaping teaspoon of the herb. Cover and steep for three minutes. Strain and sip unsweetened.

Frequency: Sip several cups throughout the day. Do not sweeten. If you find the tea bitter, add a little chamomile or mint to the mix.

■ *Greater Celandine*

Greater celandine, a slender, many-branched herb with a soft hairy covering, aids in *easing painful urination*—a common prostate symptom. It is also an excellent *aid for combatting liver problems*.

• I N S T R U C T I O N S •

GREATER-CELANDINE TEA

Preparation: Pour 1 pint freshly boiled water over 2 level teaspoons of the herb. Strain and sip. Honey may be added.

Frequency: Drink several cups throughout the day.

Other helpful herbs

Dr. Zofchak likes to blend his own tea for urinary problems: a mixture of *buchu leaves* (a bladder soother), *bearberry* (also called uva-ursi), *cubeb berries,* and *mallow*. He adds *anise* and *licorice* for taste and "balance."

An herb called *Saint-John's-wort* is useful in urinary incontinence, Zofchak said. Zofchak's prostate cures include teas made from *buchu leaves, uva-ursi,* and *saw palmetto.*

A Word of Caution

Some doctors do not believe in herbal therapies for diseases and caution patients against their use. Most doctors are not trained in the helpful uses and cures brought about by nature and are very cautious about even new technological "cure-alls."

Doctors are to a degree correct in their caution. Indeed, many herbs, though beneficial when used in carefully controlled doses can be poisonous when overused or handled incorrectly.

As Bricklin says in his *Encyclopedia of Natural Healing,* never take any herb unless you know exactly what it is and what it may do.

· CHAPTER 6

Diet as a Cure and Preventive

What goes into your body determines in a big way what comes out: good health, vigor, and long life or chronic illness, listlessness, and a shortened life span. Many physicians of different specialties have devised diet plans to suit almost every physical need. Prostate specialists are no different.

Homeostasis and Diet

Dr. Jonn Matsen, a Canadian naturopathic doctor and author, believes that not all sickness is caused by outside forces attacking body cells. He teaches that certain types of food can trigger bodily dysfunctions—including *prostatitis* and *prostatic hypertrophy*.

Matsen views the body as one cooperative unit. *Homeostasis* is a state of perfect bodily regulation, when all the body's cells work together as one. (This bodily philosophy can be found in ancient Eastern disciplines like Tao, Zen, and Hinduism.) When acute disease strikes—occasional bouts of sickness that come and go quickly—it may be the body is attempting to re-establish *homeostasis* after it has been abused, Matsen says.

The doctor says part of the American male's prostate problem is the endless variety of processed and "junk" foods the average person eats from childhood. Eating these foods shocks the digestive system, which was not designed to break down the complex chemicals added as preservatives, flavor enhancers, or coloring agents.

A body can handle an occasional dose of snack cakes and potato chips, but a regular diet of them can produce an overabundance of intestinal toxins. These overload the body's capacity to process food. Its energies go toward ridding itself of toxins rather than performing its intended task: absorbing nutrients vital to good health.

In order to rid patients of years of built-up toxins, Matsen devised a rigorous diet that hundreds of patients say brought them out of lives of fatigue and illness and back to robust health.

Starting the diet is the hardest step: permanently eliminating American staples like chocolate, coffee, tea, refined sugar, artificial sweeteners, preservatives, salt, and alcohol.

Depending on the dieter's medical needs, he next temporarily gives up certain groups of foods for several weeks. These may include peanuts, yeast, pork, shellfish, turkey, chicken, carrots, strawberries, cucumbers, walnuts, and maple syrup.

These foods are gradually reintroduced to the diet after several weeks, after the body has regained its ability to properly process food—the most important step to regaining *homeostasis*.

One of Matsen's most enthusiastic patients suffered from a colonic polyp—a growth in his lower bowel. He was overweight, suffered from high blood pressure, and suffered from frequent bouts of painful abdominal gas.

After six months on Matsen's detoxification diet, the man's weight and blood pressure were down to healthy levels. His abdominal gas pain had almost disappeared.

Those interested in learning more about the *homeostasis* diet can read Matsen's best-selling book *Eating Alive: Prevention Thru Good Digestion,* available at www.amazon.com or www.barnesandnoble.com.

Avoidance Tactics

Many doctors agree that men with prostate problems may want to avoid certain types of foods—they can interfere with medications, irritate swollen tissues, and promote urination and are sometimes linked with androgen, cholesterol, or carcinogen production.

In Chapter 3, I covered the effects of fat, cholesterol, zinc, and several other dietary items on prostate health. In support of the points I made, Dr. Peter Hill of the American Health Foundation in New York City said, "By reducing total calorie intake and substituting fruit and vegetable calories for animal calories, a high-risk prostatic cancer group was switched to a low-risk one."

Red meat has its downside. Although it is a great source of protein, it must be prepared just the right way to keep its negative effects from outweighing its benefits. Fatty cuts and most pork selections should be avoided, or at least carefully trimmed of excess fat before cooking.

Care should be taken while grilling meat: Charcoal byproducts and charring have been linked with cancer. Say no to the popular Cajun practice of "blackening" meats. Also, any meat preserved with nitrites—such as bacon, cold cuts, sausage, or smoked chops—should be avoided. Nitrites are carcinogens (cancer-linked chemicals) and are known to irritate enlarged glands.

Other items to avoid include chocolate, caffeine, pickled foods, margarine, and processed foods. Alcohol is very irritating to prostate tissue, and some men react to the flavorings in certain drinks with a type of chronic prostatitis. It's important to get enough oil in the diet, but stick to olive or safflower oils and use them sparingly. Although *unrefined flaxseed* and *pumpkin-seed oils* are recommended throughout this book, *use them only on salads*— heating them drives off their beneficial contents.

Consider Positive Foods

Instead of mulling over what you CAN'T eat, consider all the fine things you can enjoy on a sensible diet. Eat at least one large salad each day, and let its production be an outlet for your culinary creativity. By mixing colors, shapes, and shades of vegetables, fruits, nuts, and sprouts, you can enjoy your meal with all five of your senses.

One advantage to salads is their high fiber content. Researchers believe that a diet with lots of beans, fruit, and whole-wheat bread can further lower prostate risks. Men who eat more fiber get less prostate cancer, too.

Instead of eating dessert, have a piece of fresh fruit after your meal. If it is possible, stay out of the kitchen when you aren't there for a meal. Remove the salt shaker and sugar bowl from the table, so you won't be tempted. Shop for groceries *after* you've had a filling meal, so those "junk" items won't seem so appealing. Buy fresh "whole" foods whenever possible: Nutritionists say that a fresh orange or grape is twice as good for you as the juice, especially if you're trying to keep your weight under control.

As Bricklin suggests in his encyclopedia, double your buying in the store's produce section and halve your meat and deli purchases. Your prostate—and the rest of your body—will thank you.

Most people find they feel the effects of an improved diet only days after changing their eating habits. They feel more energetic and less moody, and the usual aches and pains simply don't occupy them as much. Add to this the all-important element of prevention: Study after study links a low-fat, sensible diet to a decrease in cancer risk. Those already diagnosed with cancer can use natural methods to alleviate their symptoms and sometimes even send the disease into remission – these concepts are covered in a later chapter.

But as the old saying goes, "an ounce of prevention is worth a pound of cure." The United States Department of Agriculture released in 2000 a new "food pyramid" system to measure the types and amounts of foods important to daily diets. Their recommendations are reprinted on the following pages.

FOOD GUIDE PYRAMID
A Guide to Daily Food Choices

HOW MANY SERVINGS DO YOU NEED EACH DAY?

	Women & some older adults	Children teen girls active women, most men	Teen boys & active men
Bread Group	6	9	11
Vegetable Group	3	4	5
Fruit Group	2	3	4
Milk Group	2-3*	2-3*	2-3*
Meat Group	2	2	3

* Women who are pregnant or breastfeeding

WHAT COUNTS AS ONE SERVING?

Breads, Cereals, Rice, Pasta
   1 slice of bread
   1/2 cup of cooked cereal, rice, or pasta
   1 ounce of dry cereal

Fruits
   1 medium whole fruit
   3/4 cup of juice
   1/2 cup canned fruit

Vegetables
   1/2 cup cooked vegetables
   1 cup tossed salad

Milk
   1 cup of milk
   8 ounces of yogurt
   1-1/2 to 2 ounces of cheese

Meat, Poultry, Fish, Eggs, Dry Beans, and Nuts
   3 ounces of cooked meat, poultry, or fish (3 ounces of meat is about the same size as a deck of cards)
   1/2 cup of cooked beans or 2 tablespoons of peanut butter or 1 egg counts the same as 1 ounce of meat (about 1/3 serving)

Fats, Oils, and Sweets
Use sparingly. These are foods such as salad dressings, cream, butter, margarine, sugars, soft drinks and candies. Go easy on these foods because they have a lot of calories from fat and sugars, but few nutrients.

A no-nonsense diet can be boosted by supplemental doses of *amino acids (L-glycine, L-alanine, and L-glutamine), B vitamins, zinc, vitamins A* and *E,* and a little daily dose of *unrefined flaxseed* or *pumpkin-seed oil,* both of which provide essential fatty acids needed for a healthy prostate.

Some nutrition authorities swear by the use of *prostate glandulars*—raw concentrates of glands or organs ordinarily considered problematic. Thus, many prostate-specific vitamin formulations will contain doses of ground bovine prostatic tissue— cow prostate. Some believe these tissues supply prostate-specific nutritional compounds that don't occur anywhere else. However, in light of the outbreak in Europe of mad-cow diease, extreme caution is advised when considering a supplement with any cow tissues. Many dietary supplements do not indicate where they were created, leaving open the chance for possibly contaminated bovine ingredients from those countries already affected by mad-cow disease being included in supplements found on U.S. shelves.

Nutritional Research News supplies a "label check" for men shopping for a prostate supplement at their vitamin store:

LABEL CHECK FOR PROSTATE SUPPLEMENTS

☑ Extract lipid sterolic serona repens (or saw palmetto extract)

☑ Aminoacetic acid

☑ Aminopropionic acid

☑ Alpha-aminoglutaric acid

☑ Zinc (glucinate)

☑ Vitamin B6 (Pyridoxine HCl)

☑ Vitamin A (Palmitate)

☑ Vitamin E (alpha-tocopherol succinate)

☑ Pumpkin-seed oil

☑ Cold-pressed, unrefined flaxseed oil

☑ Ginseng powder, liquid, tablets, tea, extract, or capsules

Dr. Heinrich Hergut, a Nuremberg physician, wrote an entire book on diet for men with prostate illnesses. Included in it are several of the recipes made with ingredients available in markets, co-ops, and health-food stores in the United States.

Juices and Purees

Raw food, extracted mechanically from the source, supplies rich nutrition—even for those on soft-food and non-cellulose diets.

Unreduced, fresh food is always preferable, however, and can never be completely replaced by juices. As soon as your physician allows, return to fruit and raw vegetables.

Make sure all the produce you use is well-washed. Trim off any bruises or spoiled spots. Many juicers and presses are available, from the small hand press to the motorized centerfuge. Hand presses require the fruit to be chopped first. Even when using an electric machine, it's a good idea to grate or chop apples, pears, tubers, leafy vegetables, and herbs. Those who cannot prepare juices themselves can find high-quality grape juice, other fruit juices, and vegetable juices in bottles at the health-food store.

Fruit Juices

Always serve freshly squeezed fruit juice right away. Any delay means a loss of food value. The following fruits provide delicious and wholesome juice without any admixture or extra processing: oranges, mandarin oranges, tangerines, grapefruit, apples, pears, grapes, strawberries, blueberries, currants, raspberries, peaches, apricots, sweet plums, melons, and cherries.

Many juices taste even better when mixed with one another— just check the wide variety of combinations available at the supermarket! It's best to use a citrus fruit as a "base" and add the juice of other, sweeter juices like berry, peach, apricot, or plum. For a milkshake-type texture, add a pureed banana or create a "smoothie" by using fresh, frozen fruit whirled with ice cubes in a blender or food processor.

Other additions and accents include lemon juice, unrefined sugar, honey, fruit concentrate, yogurt, buttermilk, linseed, rice and barley puree.

Vegetable Juices

Pureed vegetables should also be served fresh to preserve vitamins and minerals. The following vegetables taste fine served alone: tomatoes, turnips, beets, radishes, cabbage, celery, and all leafy, tuberous root vegetables.

Our favorite mixed vegetable juice includes equal parts of turnips, tomatoes and spinach. Other vegetables or flavorings may be added to your taste—just avoid too much salt, sugar, or other restricted items. The following provide tasty alternatives when added to your favorite vegetable-juice mix: sorrel, nettles, chives, parsley, onion, tender celery, and other herbs.

You might also try adding the following to your glass of vegetable juice: a tablespoon of yogurt or buttermilk; lemon juice; fruit-juice concentrate; and linseed, rice, or barley puree. Pureed leafy vegetables are also favored: Try white and green cabbage, endive, bok choy, or dandelions. In the springtime, gather up and add some blood-cleansing juices of nettle, sorrel, or dandelion.

If you find fresh vegetable juice too bitter or sharp-tasting, try adding a small amount of *rice or barley flour*. Stir a heaping teaspoon of flour into 7 oz. cold water; then boil for five minutes, stirring constantly. Allow the mixture to cool and add a sprinkling of the mix to each glass of vegetable juice you make. Use with care, as too much could prove constipating.

Linseed paste will also take the edge off fresh juice. It has a mildly cathartic effect on the bowels. Combine 1 tablespoon of linseeds in 7 oz. of water. Wash, and then boil 10 minutes. Sift out the hulls and allow to cool. Prepare a day's supply each morning and keep it in a thermos for blending with juices throughout the day.

Soy milk is a high-protein, mild substitute for cow's milk. Soak 1 cup of soybeans in 7 cups of water for two hours. Using the same water, boil for 20 minutes, stirring constantly. Strain juice into a pan. Add water, sugar, and 2 tablespoons of fruit sugar. Then, let cool.

Meusli: the Breakfast of Generations

The original apple meusli cereal, as first introduced by Dr. Bircher, has remained a mainstay of healthy diets through many years of treatment.

The original German recipe calls for sour, fleshy, juicy apples, such as the Jonathan, Granny Smith, and Rome varieties, but modern usage includes just about any apple you find satisfying. If late-season apples prove dry or bland, enrich the aroma by adding a little freshly grated orange peel. Some cooks "dress up" their meusli by sprinkling on a little orange juice or rose-hip puree just before serving.

D R .   B I R C H E R ' S   A P P L E   M E U S L I

1 tablespoon rolled oats, soaked for 12 hours in 3 tablespoons cold water (if using quick-cooking oats,
   simply blend together oats and water)

Add and mix to a smooth consistency:
   1 teaspoon lemon juice or orange juice
   1 tablespoon plain yogurt

a little honey

1 to 2 tablespoons water

Wash, stem and core 1/2 lb. apples. Grate the apples directly into the oat mixture, stirring occasionally so the apples do not turn brown. This makes 1 serving.

Serve immediately, garnished with a teaspoon of grated almonds. (Don't use walnuts or hazelnuts—they are too hard to digest.)

O P T I O N S :

Instead of rolled oats, use a presoaked tablespoonful of wheat germ, rice, barley, rye, buckwheat, millet, or soy flakes. To add a boost of B vitamins, add a bit of yeast flakes, available in health-food stores.

For those forbidden to consume protein, serve apple meusli with almond or sesame puree; instead of yogurt and lemon juice, use a tablespoon of ground almonds or sesame seeds and increase added water to 3 tablespoons.

Those with lactose intolerance may try the following recipe. It has a sharper taste and is less filling, but it promotes digestion and protects the liver. It is especially valuable for elderly people, because it is high in unsaturated fatty acids.

1 tablespoon rolled oats, soaked

3 tablespoons orange juice

2 tablespoons yogurt

1 tablespoon low-fat cottage cheese

1 tablespoon honey

1 tablespoon linseed oil

Mix together all the above until smooth. Grate in one large apple and one beaten banana.

Those on a *weight-gain diet* will appreciate their apple meusli with cream. Follow the basic recipe for apple meusli but beat 3 or 4 tablespoons of cream together with the lemon or orange juice.

For a special treat and an increase in your *Vitamin C intake,* make meusli with berries or small, pit-producing fruits. Don't use any sour berries!

Use 1/2 pound of washed, selected and crushed strawberries, blueberries, raspberries, blackberries, or pitted and finely chopped or food-processed, plums, peaches, or apricots.

Add the fruit to the basic meusli oat or grain mixture, instead of apples.

Try the following fruit combinations, using the same 1/2-pound proportion as you would with the apples in the recipe:

- strawberries and raspberries
- strawberries and apples
- blackberries and apples
- apples with finely cut orange or tangerine segments
- apples and bananas

Raw Vegetables

Observe the following four principals when preparing raw vegetables:

1. Process Quickly

Sun-ripened, organically grown vegetables are best, preferably grown in your own garden. Raw vegetables should be processed as little as possible and be served immediately, before wilting or loss of juice occurs. When using chopped or cut-up vegetables, serve as soon as possible to limit exposure to air.

2. Buy Quality Vegetables

Buy leafy and root vegetables that are young and tender, fully colored on all sides, and symmetrically shaped. If possible, buy produce that was grown without chemical fertilizers. This is especially important to cooks whose food is served to the ill.

3. Clean Vegetables Properly

To prevent insect infestation and infection from E-coli bacteria, scrub root vegetables under running water with a vegetable brush. If possible, make sure they were grown in a garden that does not use liquefied manure or purified plant sludge for fertilizer. Peel and immerse immediately in cold water with a little lemon juice and salt added—this preserves the bright, fresh color.

Leafy vegetables, lettuces, and cabbages should be separated from their stems, cleaned of brown or damaged areas, and allowed to soak in mildly salted water for 15 minutes—this cleanses the nooks and crannies of hidden worms and insects. Rinse each leaf separately under running water. Drain well.

Vegetables with smaller leaves, such as dandelions, Brussel sprouts, and spinach, should be carefully trimmed of tough stems and rootlets. Process these in small portions.

Tomatoes, cucumbers, and peppers, known in Germany as "fruit vegetables," require specialized processing. Cucumbers should be peeled from the center toward the outside. Trim off the ends. Small, tender cucumbers are fine if eaten unpeeled. Use only young peppers for salads. Don't peel these—simply cut them in half and remove the cores. Soak peppers in water if they taste bitter.

If there is any doubt about the farm fertilization methods used to grow the vegetables, soak them 15 minutes in a mild salt-water solution. The salt water dissolves the protein film that coats the vegetable and gives a foothold to worm eggs and vermin. Any unwelcome "dinner guests" are washed away when the food is subsequently rinsed.

Sterilize tuberous (root) vegetables by immersing the prepared vegetables in boiling water for 10 seconds. This kills germs on the outside, while leaving the insides raw.

Vegetable and fruit juices become virtually germ-free with the addition of squeezed lemon juice.

4. Harmonious Combinations

Every raw vegetable dish should, if possible, contain the "triad": a root, a fruit, and a leafy vegetable. Green-leaf vegetables are especially important for the ill. Sauces and garnishes can add the variety that relieves dietary boredom.

Neat little trimmings of herbs, radishes, young carrots, etc. can lend the raw vegetable dish a colorful, festive appearance. A serving with at least three colors enhances the beauty of the dish and contributes to the pleasure of eating. Vary combinations throughout the day, but avoid combining more than three vegetables. Try not to be too varied—even variety can get old, and excessive change can be hard on digestion.

Try preparing the following vegetables the European way:

- Lettuce, endives: serve whole leaves, or cut largest leaves in half.

- Spinach, leeks, peppers, stalk celery, fennel: cut into fine strips

- Cabbages (white, red and purple): slice leaves finely

- Small turnips, celery, beets, radishes: grate in food processor or by hand

- Jerusalem artichokes, kohlrabi, cucumber, zucchini, summer squash: slice thin

- Cauliflower: cut flower and tender parts of stem into thin slices

Sauces and Dressings for Raw Vegetables

HERB-OIL SAUCE

1 tablespoon unrefined flaxseed oil

1 teaspoon lemon juice

1 teaspoon minced onion or garlic

1 teaspoon fresh herbs, or 1 pinch dried herbs

Mix together well; use as a dip or pour over vegetable dish before serving.

MAYONNAISE SAUCE

1 beaten egg yolk

1/2 cup unrefined flaxseed oil

Add the oil a drop at a time to the egg yolk while stirring steadily with a beater. This mixture is enough for six individual portions.

For a single serving, mix together 1 tablespoon of the above yolk-oil mixture; 1 teaspoon lemon juice; a little onion or garlic, minced; and a teaspoon of herbs.

VEGETARIAN OR VEGETABLE-PROTEIN MAYONNAISE SAUCE

2 tablespoons soy flour

6 tablespoons water

Combine to a smooth batter. Alternately add the following while steadily stirring:

2 teaspoons flaxseed oil

3 tablespoons lemon juice

garlic, onion, or herbs to taste

LOW-FAT COTTAGE-CHEESE DRESSING

1/2 cup low-fat cottage cheese

1/2 teaspoon lemon juice

buttermilk as needed

Beat together to a thick sauce. Season with a little salt, chives, or parsley to taste. Use spinach or carrot juice to vary the color and taste. This is especially good served with fresh artichokes or asparagus. Try it with a raw tomato stuffed with cucumbers, celery, cauliflower, or white cabbage.

YOGURT DIP

2-3 tablespoons low-fat yogurt (plain)

several drops lemon juice

a little minced onion or garlic

fresh or dried herbs to taste

Beat ingredients together in a small bowl; serve as a dip.

A L M O N D   O R   S E S A M E   S A U C E

1 tablespoon ground almonds or pureed sesame seeds

3 tablespoons water

1 teaspoon lemon juice

onion or garlic, minced

herbs to taste

Add other ingredients slowly to almonds or sesame. This is especially good for those on diets that forbid animal protein.

C A R R O T   S A U C E

1 medium-large carrot

2 tablespoons vegetable broth

a pinch of salt

minced onion or rosemary

Place all ingredients in a mixer or food processor and puree.

V I N A I G R E T T E

1 tablespoon wheat-germ oil

1 teaspoon lemon juice

1 teaspoon water or vegetable broth

1 teaspoon boiled onion

1 to 2 sweet pickles, chopped fine

1 teaspoon diced tomato

Combine together and season with parsley, chives, and a little herbal salt.

Make Your Own Sprouts

Wheat, rye, barley, mung beans, and oats can be found at any feed store, co-op, or natural-food outlet. Sprouts made from these grains are a delicious, wholesome addition to any meal or salad.

To sprout your own grain: In the evening, wash about 2 cups of grain in a sieve under a stream of water and place it in a small bowl. Cover with water and place in a warm spot overnight.

The following morning, rinse the grain and spread it out on a plate or cookie sheet to dry. Leave in a warm spot till evening, when you should return it to its bowl and cover it again with water overnight.

Repeat the process the following day. By the fourth day, your grain will have developed sprouts of 1/4 to 1/2 inch. Snip off what you like. Take a Mason jar or other wide-mouth glass vessel and lay a water-soaked paper towel inside. Lay the jar on its side, spread the sprouted grain atop the towel, and replace the lid. Keep the jar in a warm place, keep the towel damp, and replace with more sprouted grain when the supply is low. Thus, you can keep a good, fresh vegetable and garnish on hand at all times.

Recipes for Cooked Vegetable Dishes

The first consideration when cooking vegetables is fat. For cooking, use only small amounts of sweet (unsalted) butter, sunflower oil, corn oils, and germ oils. Cold-pressed sunflower oil and olive oils are good choices for salads and sauces. They are rich in unsaturated fatty acids. Their purity makes them more easily digested than many other oils. Just remember not to heat them too quickly or intensely, as they will burn!

Soups: Recipes for One

We use quite a lot of vegetable broth in our recipes, but in a small household fresh vegetable broth cannot be prepared every day. Instead, try using ordinary tap water and an added seasoning like yeast extract (a good source of B vitamins) or vegetable bouillon. A little cream or milk improves every soup and vegetable.

VEGETABLE BROTH

1 tablespoon butter

1 onion, halved

1 stalk celery

endive

cabbage

1 stalk leek

Cut the vegetables into small pieces and steam for at least 15 minutes over low heat.

Add vegetables and butter to 2 quarts cold water. Bring to boil, reduce heat, and simmer for two hours. Season mildly with lovage or other herbs, 1/2 bay leaf, and a pinch of salt.

Pour through a sieve and serve as a clear broth.

CLEAR RICE SOUP

1/2 tablespoon butter

a little chopped onion

a little celery and leek, cut fine

2 cups vegetable broth

1 tablespoon unpolished rice

1 pinch salt

Steam all ingredients together for 45 minutes over low heat. Sieve and serve as clear broth.

For a thicker, more filling soup, sprinkle 1/2 tablespoon whole wheat or buckwheat flour over the steamed mixture. Add 1 cup of vegetable broth or water and boil another 30 minutes. Add 1/2 tablespoon milk and chopped chives to tureen before serving. May also be seasoned with marjoram, nutmeg, or caraway.

HERB SOUP

1 tablespoon whole-wheat flour

1/2 cup milk

5 cups vegetable broth, boiling

Mix the flour into half the milk and stir into the boiling broth. Simmer for 15 minutes.

Mix a tablespoon of soy flour with the remaining milk and put into the soup tureen. Beat the mixture with a hand mixer. Season with pinches of salt, lovage, marjoram, chives, nutmeg, or caraway.

S O Y   S O U P

1/2 tablespoon butter

a little chopped onion, steamed

1 tablespoon whole-wheat flour

1/2 tablespoon soy flour

1/2 tomato, peeled and diced (add just before serving)

Season with a pinch of salt, rosemary, chives, and parsley.

O A T   C R E A M   S O U P

1/2 tablespoon flour, toasted lightly in a skillet

2 tablespoons rolled oats

3 cups vegetable broth

a little celery

Combine ingredients and simmer 1 hour; strain. Add a tablespoon of butter to the tureen. Season with a pinch of salt, yeast extract, chives, or rosemary.

K A L E   S O U P

1/2 tablespoon butter

a little onion, chopped and steamed briefly

1 tablespoon leek, chopped

1 stalk celery, diced

1 large leaf of kale, soaked 12 hours in a quart of water

1 cup water

5 cups vegetable broth

Mix together in saucepan and simmer 60 to 90 minutes. Season with celery seed, salt, or ground pepper.

T O M A T O   S O U P   1

1/2 tablespoon butter

a little onion

2 tablespoons small turnips

celery

leek

1 clove garlic

a little rosemary

Cut everything finely together and steam for 10 minutes. Add one tomato, chopped. Sprinkle with 1 tablespoon whole-wheat flour. Add 3 cups vegetable broth. Simmer for 30 minutes, strain, and serve. Season with salt, cloves, chives, or a bay leaf. Also good with 1/4 cup steamed rice added.

T O M A T O   S O U P   2

4 ripe summer tomatoes, cut up, boiled, and strained

1 teaspoon lemon juice or fructose

Add one cup milk or buttermilk. Mix well; serve lukewarm or cold

P O T A T O   S O U P   W I T H   L E E K S

1/2 tablespoon butter

1/2 leek, cut in strips and steamed well

1/2 teaspoon whole-wheat flour, sprinkled over leeks and butter

3 cups vegetable broth, boiling

Combine the above. Cut in one medium potato and boil until it is soft. Season with a pinch of salt, yeast extract, and marjoram.

M I N E S T R O N E

1/2 tablespoon butter

a little onion, steamed together with 2 tablespoons leek, cut fine, and a few celery leaves

1 cup endive leaves

Combine in 4 cups of vegetable broth, season with salt, parsley, and chives, and simmer for 30 minutes. Add 1 teaspoon thyme, 1/2 clove garlic, and 1/2 cup whole-grain pasta or brown rice. Simmer together for 15 to 20 minutes. Enhance with a small pat of butter.

Sandwiches

Sandwiches are popular the world over. Served as an hors d'oeuvre for evening meals or as ready lunches on the road, this quick and easy food comes in endless variations. Men with prostate problems are usually told to stick with thin-sliced, whole-grain breads. Included here are recipes for spreads and suggested ingredients that can be arranged in all sorts of combinations to create an attractive, fresh, and appetizing appearance.

BASIC SANDWICH SPREAD

Low-fat cottage cheese or butter, stirred until frothy, and a little yeast extract, mixed in with chives, herbs, caraway seeds, or tomato puree, according to taste.

Dress up spread sandwiches with the following:

carrots | onions cut in rings | raw celery
capers | tomatoes | olives
radishes | lettuce | watercress

Boiled and Steamed Vegetables

Boiled vegetables are mild on digestion but pack plenty of vitamins. Men recovering from surgery, radiation, or chemotherapy treatments are advised to read the following carefully and put the recipes to use to ensure a quick recovery.

It is important that little salt be used to prepare all these dishes. Judicious use of spices and herbs can largely replace salt—but beware supermarket "salt substitutes." These frequently contain preservatives and flavor enhancers that could be more damaging than the real thing!

Most boiled vegetables should be served "au naturel"—that is, without dressing or garnishing. Endive, fennel, carrots, tomatoes, zucchini, beets, eggplant, and artichokes are especially good prepared this way. Avoid gas producers like cabbage, peas, beans, and spinach until your digestive system is fully recovered from your treatment or surgery.

Preparation is easy: Simply steam vegetables in or over a pan of vegetable broth or water until they are soft. Cut the vegetables into smaller pieces according to their variety.

Serve with butter, if you must, or sprinkle with herbs. Two special vegetables are artichokes and corn on the cob:

A R T I C H O K E S

Cut the stems off one or two artichokes, up close to the heads. Remove the undermost, hard leaves, and cut off the leaf tips. Halve the heads and cut out the blossoms. Wash in running water. Put 1/2 teaspoon lemon juice on the cut halves. Lay the artichokes in 2 cups water. Bring to boil and simmer 45 minutes, until artichokes are soft. Drain. Serve on a warm dish, covered with a napkin. Very good served with cottage-cheese sauce or vinaigrette.

C O R N   O N   T H E   C O B

Take one or two ears of fresh corn, shucks and silk removed. Drop them in a pan of boiling, salted water and cook for 10 minutes. Serve with fresh butter or low-fat cottage cheese. Be sure to chew each bite well or the corn will not properly digest.

S T A L K   C E L E R Y

Cut three or four stalks of celery into 3-inch pieces. Steam briefly in a frying pan. In the meantime, combine the following:

1/2 onion, chopped

1 cup vegetable broth

2 tablespoons milk or a little lemon juice

a pinch of salt

Simmer together until tender, about 30 minutes. Combine with celery stalks in frying pan; season with celery seed and yeast extract.

STEAMED CELERY

1/2 tablespoon butter

1/2 onion, steamed briefly

3 or 4 stalks celery with tops, cut into small slices and steamed

Add 2 cups of vegetable broth and, simmer 30-45 minutes until celery is tender. Season with marjoram or lemon juice.

CELERY SECTIONS

1 stalk celery

Cut into quarters and boil until tender in the following:

1/2 cup milk

1/2 cup water

a pinch of salt

Cut into wafer-thin slices and serve like flakes on a hot serving plate. Cover with toasted cracker crumbs and melted butter.

CHOPPED SPINACH

Carefully select four to six deep-green spinach leaves. Chop them up; discard any thick stems; wash well. Boil briskly a short while in 2 cups of vegetable broth. Reserve broth.

In a separate container, steam together briefly a little chopped onion and

a little garlic. Remove from heat and add 1 tablespoon flour, the water poured off the spinach, above and a pinch of salt. Simmer all together for 15 minutes. Add the spinach and heat through. Season with peppermint leaves, sage, and fresh butter. Just before serving, add 1 cup finely chopped raw spinach leaves.

*Do not serve spinach to patients with diarrhea.

GREEN PEAS

1/2 tablespoon butter

a little onion, lightly steamed

3/4 cup green peas

1 cup vegetable broth

a pinch of salt

Combine ingredients in frying pan; boll for 10 minutes. Season with parsley, chives, or marjoram.

*Peas should be served only to those who can tolerate them. Do not serve them to patients plagued with flatulence!

RED BEETS

Simmer 2 cups red beets for two hours. Peel and cut into thin slices. Melt 1/2 tablespoon butter and add to the beets. Pour in 1/2 cup vegetable broth and steam for 15 minutes. Add a pinch of salt and 1/2 tablespoon flour before serving. Season with lemon, caraway, lemon balm, nutmeg, parsley, or a little garlic.

STEWED TOMATOES

Blanch four or five fresh tomatoes in boiling water and peel. Place in frying pan with a tablespoon of oil, 1/2 tablespoon butter, 1/2 onion, and a sprinkling of fruit sugar. Steam together, breaking up tomatoes as they cook and thicken. Add a little minced garlic and a tablespoon of cornstarch for binding and then a pinch of chopped parsley. Other herbs such as rosemary, basil, chives, or marjoram, may be sprinkled over the tomatoes when they are served.

STUFFED TOMATOES

Cut the tops off two or three tomatoes. Hollow them out, chop the pulp, and mix with 1 teaspoon of uncooked rice per tomato. Replace in the tomato shell. Season to taste with rosemary, basil, onion, or garlic. Put 1/2 teaspoon butter atop each and replace the tops. Bake at 325 F for 30 minutes. Sprinkle with toasted crumbs and serve with a cup of soup.

TOMATOES WITH SCRAMBLED EGGS

1 or 2 tomatoes, cut up and stewed

1 large egg or 1 portion egg substitute

1 tablespoon cream

a pinch of salt

Mix together all ingredients and scramble in a small frying pan. Season with chives or garlic.

RED CABBAGE

1/2 tablespoon butter

1/2 onion, chopped

2 cups red cabbage, sliced fine

Steam all three ingredients together for 15 minutes and add the following:

1/2 tablespoon lemon juice

1/2 apple, sliced thin

1/2 tablespoon rice

1 1/2 cups vegetable broth

Steam all ingredients over low heat for 1 to 1 1/2 hours. Spread on a baking sheet, coat with butter and broil briefly.

Garnish before serving with mixture of 1/2 cup grape juice or fruit juice; a peeled, sliced apple; a little butter; and a pinch of salt.

*Those with a tendency to flatulence should avoid cabbage dishes.

TENDER EGGPLANT

1 medium eggplant, washed, peeled, and diced

1 small onion, chopped

Steam together with a pinch of salt and a pat of butter for 25 minutes. Serve with a cup of broth and a pinch of salt. Garnish with tomato halves or stewed tomatoes.

STEAMED OR BOILED VEGETABLE SALADS

Carrots, small turnips, beets, beans, and cauliflower are especially suited for these salads. Steam the vegetables in water or vegetable stock until tender. Cut into small slices, cubes, or strips. Dress with mayonnaise sauce, herb-oil dressing, or vinaigrette. Use chopped herbs for seasoning.

POTATO SALAD

2 medium potatoes, boiled, peeled, and sliced

1/2 cup hot vegetable broth.

1 tablespoon flaxseed or sunflower oil

1 tablespoon lemon juice

1/2 tablespoon chopped onion

a pinch of salt

Pour vegetable broth over sliced, boiled potatoes

and let them stand for a few minutes. Combine oil, lemon juice, chopped onion, and salt and beat together well. Pour dressing mixture over potatoes and let stand a while before serving. Season with parsley, dill, sour cream, mustard, or celery seed. You may also enjoy this with 1/4 of a cucumber and some chives grated in.

RICE SALAD

1 cup unpolished brown rice

2 cups water

1 tablespoon sunflower oil

1/2 tablespoon lemon juice

1/2 tablespoon onions

1/2 tomato

chives, parsley, and basil to taste

lettuce leaves (or pastry shells)

Cook 1 cup brown, unpolished rice in 2 cups water. Rinse briefly and allow to cool. Beat together 1 tablespoon sunflower oil and 1/2 tablespoon lemon juice.

Fold in 1/2 tablespoon onions and 1/2 tomato, diced fine. Spice with chives, parsley, and basil. Mix in with the rice. Serve over lettuce leaves or pastry shells.

Potato Dishes

POTATOES IN THEIR JACKETS

Three or four small potatoes (red or yellow are especially good), brushed and washed.

Place in colander or pan with perforated double boiler. Fill pot with water up to the level of the perforated pan and add a pinch of salt. Put the potatoes inside, cover, and boil 30 or 40 minutes.

BAKED POTATOES

Two or three potatoes, brushed and washed. Scratch the skin on the upper side of each potato. Paint each with a little oil and bake 30 to 40 minutes at 350 degrees F. on a greased baking tray. To serve, split each potato open and insert a pat of butter.

PARSLEY POTATOES

Take two or three potatoes, peeled, quartered, and steamed. Melt a tablespoon of butter. Mix in a tablespoon of chopped parsley and a pinch of salt. Pour over hot potatoes and serve.

COTTAGE CHEESE POTATOES

2 or 3 potatoes, baked according to above directions

Mix together:

1/2 cup low-fat cottage cheese

1 to 2 tablespoon milk

chives or caraway seeds

a pinch of salt

Stir ingredients together and use as a topping on the hot potatoes.

CARAWAY POTATOES

two to three medium-large potatoes, washed and cut in half lengthwise.

Mix a teaspoon of caraway seeds with a pinch of salt. Dab the cut surface of the potatoes in the caraway salt mixture. Place face-down on a greased metal baking sheet. Paint tops with oil and bake 45 minutes at 350 degrees F. For Sesame Potatoes, simply substitute sesame seeds for the caraway.

BOUILLON POTATOES

Boil two or three potatoes. In a separate pan, boil 2 cups vegetable broth, a pinch of salt, and small cubes of leftover carrot, leek, celery, or turnips. Boil until vegetables are soft; spread over the potatoes before serving. Season with thyme, bay leaf, or parsley.

MASHED POTATOES

4 potatoes, peeled, cut up, steamed or boiled until tender, and drained.

Add a little water or milk to potatoes; then pass through a potato press or process with a masher or food processor. Add 2 1/2 tablespoons of butter and 1/2 cup milk to potatoes; stir until foamy. Season with chopped marjoram, caraway, dried tomato, or ground pepper. Serve on a hot dish. Some European cooks like to sculpt the potatoes with a hot, wet knife before serving.

POTATO SLICES WITH SPINACH

1 large potato, peeled and cut lengthwise into quarter-inch slices. Boil in 2 cups vegetable broth until tender.

Lay them in a single layer on a buttered baking sheet. Take a cup of chopped spinach (recipe above); layer over potatoes. Dot with butter. Season with parsley, chives, and nutmeg. Broil dish briefly at 450 degrees F.

Grain or Cereal Dishes

RISOTTO

1/2 cup risotto pasta

1/2 cup unpolished rice

Boil together in 2 1/2 cups of vegetable broth or water for 30-40 minutes.

Mix in a pinch of salt and a pat of butter just before serving; sprinkle with parsley or rosemary.

TOMATO RICE

1/2 cup unpolished rice

1 1/2 cups vegetable broth

Simmer over low heat for 30 to 40 minutes. Add 1 tomato, peeled and cubed.

Mix in a pat of butter and a pinch of salt; season with rosemary, basil, or nutmeg.

RICE WITH SPINACH

1 cup spinach, coarsely cut

3/4 cup unpolished rice

3 cups hot vegetable broth

Simmer these together for 30 minutes. Add a pinch of salt and season with basil, peppermint, or parsley.

RICE PUDDING WITH TOMATOES

3/4 cup unpolished rice

3 cups vegetable broth

1 tablespoon minced carrots, leeks, or celery

Simmer all ingredients together for 30 minutes and set aside. Cut three fresh tomatoes into slices. Layer pudding and tomatoes in a buttered baking pan. Sprinkle with parsley, a little salt, and dots of butter. Bake 10 minutes at 325 degrees F.

Sauces

Serve these sauces warm, over rice, pasta, or grain dishes

TOMATO SAUCE

Cut up two or three tomatoes and steam until tender; strain. Add a little herbal salt and some oregano plus a little fresh butter or a tablespoon of milk.

HERBAL SAUCE

Warm 1/2 tablespoon butter. Sprinkle a tablespoon of flour over the warmed butter and stir. Add 1 1/2 cups milk all at once, stir. Add 1/2 cup vegetable broth and simmer 20 minutes. Season with chervil, basil, or tarragon.

Vegetable Roast for Special Occasions

This is not a "dietary food" like fresh fruit, vegetables, salads, or whole-grain dishes but it is incomparably more nutritious than meat roasts. When serving, always present a raw vegetable course first followed by a soup or salad before serving the "roast"—in this case, an old German recipe. Caraway potatoes are traditionally served with this dish.

CARLSBAD PATTIES
(FOUR SERVINGS)

Take 2 1/2 cups whole rolled oats and boil to a thick paste in water or broth: Add 1 large onion, cut into pieces and roasted until yellow. Combine 1 tablespoon butter, parsley, celery salt, marjoram and a tablespoon of soy flour.

Mix into oatmeal. Stir well and then grate in two or three boiled potatoes. A stiff dough will form. Roll pinches of the dough into 1/4-inch thick patties. Dredge them in whole-wheat flour. Coat a frying pan with oil, lay in the patties and bake them for 1 hour at 350 degrees F.

Sweet Dishes to Serve 4

Too many sweets and pastries are especially bad for elderly or recovering patients, because sugar promotes fermentation and flatulence. Sugar robs the body of B vitamins, which are especially important to aging tissues. Instead of using commercial white sugar, try using fruit concentrates, honey, or fructose.

BERRIES AND YOGURT

Select and wash your choice of strawberries, blueberries, white currants or raspberries: about 1 pint Mix some fruit concentrate or lemon juice into a pint of plain yogurt, place into single serving bowls or compotes. Decorate the top of the yogurt with the berries.

FRUIT CREAM

1 pint berries, oranges, or melons, cut up

1 pint low-fat cottage cheese

Mix fruit with low-fat cottage cheese, strain away extra liquid, add a little lemon juice or fruit concentrate, mix, and serve.

VANILLA CREAM

2 cups milk

1 vanilla bean, halved lengthwise

Put both into a saucepan and slowly bring milk to a boil. Stir 2 tablespoons cornstarch together with a little cool milk; stir into the hot pan with a tablespoon of fructose. Bring to a boil again; then allow to cool.

FRUIT SALAD

To make the syrup combine 1 cup of water with 1/4 cup honey and boil. Allow to cool. Add 1 cup grape juice or other light fruit juice. Set aside.

Combine seasonal fruits to make 4 or 5 cups total: try apricots, peaches, melons, apples, pears, cherries, or berries. Cut the fruit into small chunks and put into the syrup. Chill and then serve in small dishes—This is also attractive served in seeded melon halves.

APPLE SAUCE

Boil 2 pounds apples, stemmed, peeled, and cut up in 2 quarts of water until soft; then strain. Mix in a little fructose, cinnamon, and lemon zest. Serve warm or cold. If a smooth apple sauce is desired, whirl the mixture in a blender or food processor before serving.

BLUEBERRY SPREAD

This dish is good for diarrhea sufferers.

Boil 1 pint of washed blueberries in a quart of water for 5-10 minutes. Add a little fructose and a tablespoon of flour and bring to a boil. Dot top of the mixture with a tablespoon of butter. Pour over toasted bread or bread cubes.

STRAWBERRY SMOOTH

1 cup strawberry slices, washed and trimmed

1 1/2 tablespoons fruit concentrate or fructose

1 tablespoon low fat cottage cheese

1 tablespoon yogurt

Mix together all ingredients; strain through a sieve. Serve in cups decorated with berry halves. Don't limit yourself to strawberries: other berries in season work well, too.

STRAWBERRY OR RASPBERRY CREAM

1 pint berries

1 cup milk

1 vanilla bean, split lengthwise

Mix together, strain, and bring to a boil. Serve warm.

BAKED STUFFED APPLES

4 large or 8 small apples, cored, with grooves cut in the skins

Optional filling:

2 tablespoons raisins or currants

1 tablespoon cream

fructose or honey

1 grated lemon peel

Mix together all filling ingredients, put inside apples, and place on a baking pan. Drizzle with melted butter; fill each apple core within 1/4 inch of the top with fruit juice.

Bake at 325 degrees F for 30 minutes. (You may also bake the apples without the stuffing.)

LEMON-RICE PUDDING

Boll together 1 quart water, the juice of one lemon, diced lemon peel, a pinch of salt, and a dribble of honey.

Add 1 1/2 cups of unpolished rice, reduce heat, and simmer, covered, for 30 minutes. Remove from heat and allow to cool. Pour into a Jell-O mold or tube pan and refrigerate. Serve cold.

COTTAGE-CHEESE PUDDING

Combine 1/4 cup butter and 4 tablespoons of flour in a pan; brown the flour. Add 1 1/2 cups milk and boil several minutes.

Mix in a pint of low-fat cottage cheese, 1 beaten egg, 1/4 cup fruit concentrate, 1/2 cup raisins, and a grated lemon peel. Pour mixture into a

Jell-O mold or tube pan, bake at 325 degrees F for 30 or 40 minutes. Serve warm.

Health Teas

CHAMOMILE TEA

Infuse a tablespoon of chamomile in a cup of boiling water. Chamomile tea eases stomach pain and, cleanses and calms the digestive system. It's also used for enemas and douches.

PEPPERMINT TEA

Infuse a tablespoon of peppermint leaves in a cup of boiling water. Peppermint tea calms the stomach and stimulates bile production to speed digestion. This is a popular "pleasure beverage" and makes delicious iced tea.

ROSE-HIP TEA

Rose hips are available from your health-food store or your neighborhood rosebush. Soak 2 or 3 table-spoons of minced or powdered rose hips and skins in 3 quarts of water for 12 hours. Simmer the liquid slowly for 30 to 45 minutes, then strain. This tea is lightly diuretic (water-shedding) and stimulates digestion. Its lightly tart flavor makes it a nice complement to meals.

LINSEED TEA

Boil 1 tablespoon of linseed (flaxseed) in 2 cups of water for 7 to 10 minutes. The tea is cleansing, lightly laxative, and helps the body to digest raw fruit juices.

What Can I Do? Exercise!

It is ironic that prostate sufferers so often find themselves passive recipients of medical treatments. When a disease strikes so close to the "heart" of his manhood, the average man feels he must take an active role in its resolution.

Happily, activity itself can aid in recovery and prevention of prostatitis, prostate hypertrophy, and sometimes prostate cancer. Physicians of cultures throughout the world have developed plans that men themselves work at on a day-to-day basis at home, which enables the patients to participate in their own cure.

Men whose problems are not severe can use no-nonsense approaches to improved prostate health. One way is to use the bathroom frequently. "Holding on" simply irritates and stretches the bladder and can worsen a latent problem.

Going on long car trips can be a trial for a prostate patient, as travel frequently increases the urge to "go." Before leaving on a journey, cut back on caffeine and salty food, which move liquids quickly through the system. As inconvenient as it may be, stop frequently to empty your bladder.

Men who experience *dysuria*, or *"dribbling,"* problems, can benefit from Kegel exercises, which constitute an internal workout that strengthens the muscles in the lower pelvis. Popularized by proponents of natural childbirth and named for the doctor who discovered its benefits, this squeezing motion can help men with weak urine streams better control their bladder muscles.

• INSTRUCTIONS •

KEGEL EXERCISE

To do a Kegel exercise, simply squeeze the muscles you'd normally use to hold back or stop a stream of urine. Hold for a count of three and then release for a count of three. Repeat 25 times, three times a day. The "workout" is perfectly silent and still and can be done in the midst of a day's work without notice or undue exertion.

Along with a change in diet, *exercise* is the easiest, least-expensive habit a man can develop to keep his prostate healthy.

Exercise doesn't necessarily mean strenuous weightlifting or long hours of racquet swinging. The one form of exercise that is far superior to any other for prostate maintenance is *walking*.

The splendid aspect of walking is its simplicity. No fancy, expensive equipment is needed, and there's no need to visit a personal trainer for "walking lessons." Anyone who is not handicapped can walk. It promotes togetherness and conversation, making it an ideal workout for couples. Regular evening walks may even put some romance back into your life!

If prostate health and perhaps your future sexual health aren't impetus enough to get you off the sofa and walking around the block, perhaps these facts will help.

Daily walking, even for just 30 minutes, has the following effects on the human body.

1. It lowers your chances of having a heart attack.

In a continuing study of Harvard University alumni, researchers find that men who burn at least 2,000 calories a week walking or doing other moderate exercise have a 28 percent lower death rate from cardiac problems than those who do little or no exercise. This and other studies show that a regular walking program lowers a man's blood pressure and his resting heart rate.

2. It lowers levels of artery-clogging blood fats.

This works hand in hand with a lowered risk of heart attack, and also benefits the arteries that supply blood to the genitals and enable a man to get an erection. Men whose arteries are clogged with cholesterol fats may not have sufficient blood flow to create a firm erection.

Walking lowers these blood fats that narrow arteries and increases levels of HDL, the "good cholesterol" that fights fatty buildup.

3. It controls body weight.

Walking increases your body's metabolism, which burns calories. Exercise increases the conversion of fat cells to energy and builds muscle tissue, which in turn burns more calories. Regular walking also tends to curb one's appetite.

4. It improves one's mental outlook.

A good workout releases *endorphins*, natural mood-elevating brain chemicals. Walking can actually put you in a good mood. A recent study showed that it is more effective than tranquilizers at relieving anxiety.

5. It relieves back pain.

Walking strengthens and tones muscles that stabilize the spine. Unlike jogging, it puts little stress on the spinal disks and knee and ankle joints. In fact, walking puts less stress on your spine than sitting does!

6. It increases energy.

Instead of eating a candy bar when you need a quick burst of energy, try taking a 10-minute walk. Dr. Robert Mayer, a professor at California State University, headed a study that found a walk as short as 10 minutes not only produces extra energy but also produces a sudden "burst" of energy that outlasts the "power boost" of a candy bar. Walkers also display less muscle tension than their candy-munching counterparts, Thayer found.

Chuck N. says he's a living example of the benefits of walking. When he was a young man, Chuck didn't have a car. He walked to work, to dates, and to the store and back, never even thinking twice about "exercise." He had little choice.

As he grew older, Chuck continued to walk—then to work and appointments. By then he had a car of his own, but he used it only for longer trips.

Today, Chuck is a strapping, healthy 95-year-old. He's never had a problem with his prostate, he says, and continues to walk every day.

Massage and Prostate Problems

One of the best ways to soothe an irritated prostate is to massage it. Many urologists bring patients needed relief by stroking the gland with a gloved finger. The doctor accesses the gland anally and then presses down on the prostate, beginning at the top and working toward the bottom. This empties the gland of excess secretions and reduces its size enough to provide temporary relief. It works by stimulating circulation to the gland, which in turn reduces inflammation.

Many doctors advise patients like Howard H. to massage their own prostate glands. Howard visited his doctor because he couldn't urinate—his prostate had swollen to twice its normal size. His hips ached, and a intermittent fever sometimes reached 101 degrees F.

The doctor massaged Howard's prostate and then advised him to buy some rubber finger cots at the drugstore. Finger cots are rubber tubes that fit snugly over a finger. With this equipment, Howard continued his treatment at home. (Some men prefer to use less-expensive condoms, some of which are manufactured with a lubricant.)

INSTRUCTIONS

PROSTATE MASSAGE

Consult your doctor before beginning this procedure: Improper massage may further irritate your prostate. This is best done in a sitting position, usually on a toilet seat, or standing, with one foot on a chair.

Cover your index finger with a cot. Insert the finger about 1 1/2 inches into your rectum. Very gently stroke the rounded shape of the prostate just as your doctor does, starting at the top and working toward the bottom. The massage may be done every other day or even daily, depending on your condition and doctor's advice.

Reflexology

Reflexology is a system of physical culture that is based on therapeutic massage. By massaging various reflex points of the body, you not only eliminate pain in the region being massaged but also release healing energy throughout the body.

You may be familiar with these reflex points if you've heard of acupuncture. Practitioners of this ancient Chinese healing method teach that these points are energy junctions that relay and reinforce energy along the body's "meridian lines," which send vital energy through the organs via the nervous system.

Reflexologists don't use needles, however. They use their hands and fingers to massage the reflex points, releasing endorphins into the body tissues. These "feel-good" neurotransmitters suppress pain and produce a calming or even euphoric effect on the body. It's the same chemical that produces the long-distance runner's "high."

Reflexologist Mildred Carter, author of the book *Body Reflexology: Healing at Your Fingertips*, writes that men can use this massage system to alleviate prostate symptoms. Dale L., 22, avoided prostate surgery by using reflexology.

After Dale's BPH diagnosis, he visited several doctors an specialists, seeking a nonsurgical answer to his dilemma. They all recommended prostate surgery, but Dale felt he was too young for that.

After reading up on *reflexology*, Dale began stimulating the "reflex buttons" on his wrists (see diagram).

After only two weeks of regular massage, Dale's prostate problems were gone, including a bad case of nocturia—the need to urinate frequently at night. He wrote, "I feel like I should have been feeling all these years—energetic—and I have a new lease on life. I feel better now than I can remember feeling ever before in my life."

MASSAGING REFLEXES OF THE HAND

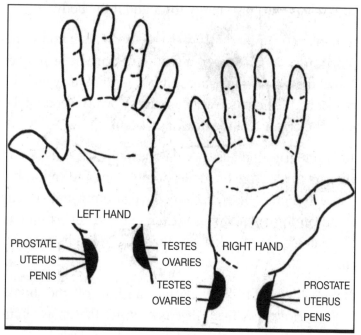

Nerve centers associated with the prostate are located directly beneath the thumbs about an inch below the wrist.

To make use of this Oriental cure, simply massage the same area on both wrists several times a day. If there is tenderness or pain, continue to gently massage. This indicates a problem with the organ or gland being treated, Carter says.

Other prostate-related reflex buttons are located on the outside of the feet, below and slightly behind the protrusion of the ankle bone. Massaging here will also bring prostate relief.

MASSAGING REFLEXES OF THE FOOT

If neither of these points works for you after two weeks of massage, get to the root of the problem. Massage the area around the base of the penis with your fingertips. If this band of muscle feels hard to the touch, massage it until the hardness vanishes and the tissue is pliable as Carter advises.

Internal Exercises: Move Your Chi Around

Over 2,500 years ago, the Chinese developed *Tao* (rhymes with "plow")—a philosophy of serenity and longevity for one's mind, body, and spirit as well as for society. "Chi" is a word for the body's natural healing energy. Integral to Tao-and Buddhism-is a system of fitness called "tai chi." Its elegant, dancelike movements are frequently portrayed in documentaries and martial-arts demonstrations. I don't intend to teach tai chi but only touch on an unseen aspect of its discipline: the internal exercise.

Dr. Stephen T. Chang, author of *The Complete System of Self-healng: Internal Exercises*, writes of the benefits of putting the body's natural healing energy to work on specific internal organs and glands.

For clarity's sake, I will explain a basic philosophy shared by Tao, Zen, Hinduism, and other Eastern religions—the existence of several nerve centers, what the Indians call *chakras*, laid in a pathway "from top to tail." When the body is healthy, energy can travel freely from one *chakra* to another, finally reaching the pineal gland, or "head chakra," the seat of spirituality.

When practiced regularly, internal exercises balance the body's energy level and promote more effective functions in major organs. Thus is the body better able to heal its injuries, adjust to environmental changes, correct abnormalities and fight disease.

Internal exercises can help your body heal prostatic problems and improve your spirituality and sex life too, Tao experts assert. The best prostate exercise is called the *Deer Exercise*. It is said to not only prevent but also reverse *prostatitis* and *prostatic hypertrophy*.

Contemplating nature is an important element of Tao practice, and the sages who developed the internal exercises reflect this contemplation in the names they give the practices. Three long-lived animals, the deer, turtle, and crane inspired series of exercises the sages derived from observing them.

The deer was admired for his strong sexual and reproductive powers. The wise men noticed that dominant stags exercised their anal muscles every time they twitched their tails, and an exercise was born.

INSTRUCTIONS

DEER EXERCISE

Stage 1: Rub the palms of your hands together to bring your body's energy to your hands.

Place the palm of your right hand over your testicles, completely covering them but not squeezing. Place the palm of your left hand on your pubic bone—about an inch below your navel. Move your left hand slowly in a clockwise circle 81 times, exerting only slight pressure on the pubis.

Rub your palms together again.

Reverse the position of your hands, placing your left hand over your testicles and your right hand on your pubis—the bony ridge at the base of your belly. Repeat the 81 circles but in a counterclockwise direction.

Concentrate on the energy moving between your two palms. This is extremely important, Chang asserts, as it unifies body and mind.

If you get an erection during the exercise, take the hand from your testicles and place it over the base of your

CONTINUED ON NEXT PAGE

DEER EXERCISE, CONTINUED

penis. Press down sharply while massaging the pubis area with the other hand. This inhibits blood flow to the penis and maximizes energy build up within your internal sex glands.

Stage 2: Stand with your hands in the stage 1 position. Tighten the muscles of your anus, drawing them upward and inward. It should feel as if air is being drawn into your rectum. Tighten as much as possible and hold this position as long as it is comfortable.

Stop and rest for a moment; then repeat the anal contraction as many times as is comfortable. (if this reminds you of the Kegel Exercise explained above, you are correct—it works out the same muscle group.) While you squeeze, concentrate on the sensations traveling along the pathway between your belly, back, throat, and head—the chi flowing along your internal pathway. Don't force this sensation with mental images. It will occur naturally and last for only a fraction of a second.

At first, it may be difficult to hold the contraction for longer than a few seconds. After several weeks, though, there should be a noticeable improvement. To test the effectiveness of the *Deer Exercise*, try to stop your urine stream when you use the bathroom through use of anal contractions. If you can stop the flow—say thank you to the Tao masters!

During the Deer Exercise, the tightening anal muscles gently massage the prostate gland. That gland, in turn secretes endorphins, those friendly "feel-good" chemicals. Other advantages include increased sensitivity around the pubis and penis, which may help with impotence and premature ejaculation. Moreover, the Tao masters believed the *Deer Exercise* enlarges the bulb at the penis' tip, which gives a man more pleasurable intercourse.

For maximum benefit, do the *Deer Exercise* twice each day, morning and night.

Another simple Chinese exercise designed to increase circulation to the sex glands is described below.

INSTRUCTIONS

SEXUAL GLANDS EXERCISE

Sit on the floor and bend your knees so that the soles of your feet touch in front of your body.

Rub the bottoms of your feet together until they are warm and then put them together.

Rub your toes with your fingers until they are warm. With your feet held together, draw your heels up toward your pelvis as close as is comfortable. Hold your toes with your hands and, using your elbows, press your knees toward the floor.

Rub the insides of your thighs with your palms. Start at the knees and continue massaging upward to the inner pelvis. Repeat this massage seven times.

Gently pummel your inner thighs with your fists to stimulate blood circulation and energy in your legs and sexual organs. Continue the exercise as long as comfort allows.

Answers From India

Yoga is another program brought to us from far away in space and time. Physicians are now accepting this 5,000-year-old Indian therapy for the curative physical-therapy program it is.

According to doctors at the Yoga Research Laboratory at Lonavia, India, one simple Yoga "pose" is especially beneficial to prostate sufferers: It is called the *Kneeling Pose*. Yoga's *Mudra Pose* requires a bit more flexibility. It increases circulation to the genital area. It also works the colon muscles and relieves constipation—but don't try these exercises on a full stomach, or if you have arthritis or other problems with your joints.

INSTRUCTIONS

YOGA'S KNEELING POSE

Sit on your heels on the floor, your back straight. Relax. SLOWLY separate your feet and let your bottom sink between them until it touches the floor. Repeat 15 times or more, being careful not to twist your knee joints.

YOGA'S MUDRA POSE

Sit cross-legged on the floor. Let out your breath, and slowly lean forward until your forehead touches the floor in front of you. Reach behind your back and grasp the wrist of one hand in the other. Hold for a count of 5, inhale, and slowly rise back to a sitting position. Repeat for up to 15 minutes.

More Sex

Other suggested therapies are practiced worldwide: The most popular is espoused by Stephen N. Rous, M.D., author of *The Prostate Book*. His suggested cure for nonbacterial prostate problems is more sex.

Rous reasons that a decrease in sexual release can cause ejaculate to accumulate in the prostate to the point of pain. Indeed, many men—especially younger ones—complain of this mysterious "blue balls" ailment when their partners cannot or will not cooperate with their sexual wishes.

Increased sex is a favorite therapy for many when prostate symptoms flare up—I won't include instructions for it here! But be sure to discuss with your doctor any symptom that returns regularly or impedes sexual performance.

Baths: Circulizers and Sitz Baths

For almost 40 years, Europeans have treated circulatory and vascular problems with a method that makes use of the "consensual-reaction" theory, also known as the *Dastre-Moratsche* reaction.

This reaction is illustrated best by an old adage: "Get cold feet, get a cold." A second look at Mom's warnings about getting your feet wet on a chilly day may hold scientific water: A shock to the cold receptors in the feet can effectively lower temperatures in a patient's mouth, sinuses, and outer ear canals—which may just make him more susceptible to catching a cold.

Doctors Dastre and Moratsche put a reverse spin on these findings and came up with a warming footbath therapy that gets good results for thousands of European users.

Their bath unit, marketed as the F-S Circulizer in the United States, uses a slowly rising temperature and several healing herbs to expand the tiny capillaries in the soles of the feet. As the water temperature rises, the blood vessels in the feet expand to maximum, starting a chain reaction of dilation throughout the circulatory system.

Extensive testing has shown the circulizer to be effective in dealing with *impotency, colds, flu, bronchitis, angina, bladder irregularities, asthma, migraine headaches, dizziness, insomnia, arthritis, prostate problems, osteoporosis, low and high blood pressure, varicose veins, lupus,* and many more ailments.

This treatment is especially helpful for men whose prostates aren't the only organs they have problems with and whose medical conditions preclude surgery.

One 83-year-old subject had a heart condition. His advanced age, coupled with the cardiac problem and a prostate the size of a chicken egg, made him turn to the circulizer as a last resort. Even the weakest heart isn't endangered by a footbath, so his doctor consented.

Four weeks later, the same doctor expressed amazement at his patient's marked improvement. The elderly man's prostate had returned to normal size.

Sitz Baths

Many doctors recommend prostate patients take hot *sitz baths* to shrink their swollen glands. Naturopathic physician Paavo Airola frequently prescribed them to his patients.

The water should be as hot as you can stand. About 8 inches of water will usually be enough; you should sit in the bath with your knees drawn up toward your chest. Stay in the water for

10 to 15 minutes; repeat two or three times a week. In most cases, the hot water alone provides relief from inflammation. But those with acute problems may want to add some chamomile tea to the bath.

INSTRUCTIONS

CHAMOMILE TEA

Preparation: Boil one pint of water and add 1 ounce of chamomile blossoms. Cover the pot tightly and steep for 10 to 12 minutes; don't let vapor escape with the medicinal qualities.

Strain out the leaves and pour the liquid into the hot bath water.

A Specialized Exercise Program for Men

Many natural-health adherents have discovered a low-impact exercise method that is proven to improve cardiopulmonary fitness and condition the body systems that serve the prostate gland.

This device was used by former President Ronald Reagan during his White House years, when he couldn't get outdoors to exercise. Studies by NASA and the U.S. Air Force found the rebounder exerciser 68 percent more effective than jogging, providing measurable reductions in body fat and high improvement in fitness levels.

The *rebounder*, or mini trampoline, provides a stress-free way to work out in your own home. Engaging in rebound aerobics allows you to save your joints while improving your cardio health and weight resistance. It is a great tool for men who want to start a fitness program but need to start out slowly.

REBOUNDING:
The Exercise of Choice

No matter what your age, rebounding helps you regain youthful vitality.

Rebounding exercisers trace their origins to the trampoline, a bouncy platform invented in 1936 and used extensively by athletes and trainers through the World War II era to develop coordination, timing, and flexibility. Pole-vaulters, gymnasts, wrestlers, soccer players, and skiers still make good use of trampolines in their training programs.

Trampolines became popular in schools and fitness facilities during the 1950s and 1960s—kids enjoyed the high flying and bouncing so much they didn't realize how much exercise they were getting. Unfortunately, a lack of supervision and abuse by daredevils gave the trampoline an early exit from public schools.

The first modern *rebounders* appeared in the 1970s; they were little more than small trampolines. These apparatuses developed through time; sturdy handrails, stiffer springs, and a more even tension were added. The mini trampolines became an effective training machine.

Rebounding has become the exercise of choice for many Americans who previously hesitated to jump into the fitness craze. A jogging or walking motion on a *rebounder* provides all the exercise of normal motion without the steady pounding experienced by runners, joggers, and walkers, making it an ideal exerciser for diabetics and those recovering from injuries or surgery. The firm "bounce-back" of the polypropylene mat builds endurance levels and lower-body muscles but pampers joints and tendons.

Many folks new to exercise are shy about working out in a gym or health club. Others don't have more than a few minutes each day to give to exercise, or can't leave their home or office for the time it takes to work out.

Rebounding is the ideal answer to all these dilemmas. No special wardrobe, membership fee, transportation, or time demands are required—you can "bound" in the privacy of your home, whatever the weather, in your undershorts if you like! And the unit folds easily into a carrying case for easy storage and travel.

Dr. James R. White wrote that rebounding for a sufficient amount of time each week changes and improves every cell in the body, increasing endurance, aerobic capacity, and cardiovascular health.

The key to rebounding is gravity, putting nature's resistance to work for you. Bouncing isn't necessary. Even those recovering from serious illness can put the bounder to good use by sitting on the platform, grasping the stability bar, and pulling their bodies upward by their arms.

For more information on this unique exercise program and where to purchase your own *rebounder*, contact the American Institute of Reboundology; tel. 1-888-464-JUMP, web site: www.healthbounce.com.

· C H A P T E R 8 ·

Prostate Cancer
The Big C and Treatments

Prostate cancer is a disease most men know little about—and would rather not think about. But like it or not, prostate-cancer awareness is growing.

A prostate-cancer screening booth was set up at the 1992 Republican National Convention, at the urging of former Republican leader of the U.S. Senate and prostate-cancer survivor Bob Dole. A rash of celebrity deaths from prostate cancer—actors Telly Savalas, Don Ameche, and Bill Bixby; musician Frank Zappa; and entertainment mogul Steve Ross—served to launch the "quiet killer" into the feature pages of *Newsweek* and *Time* and into the national consciousness.

In more recent years prostate-cancer awareness programs have sprung up on both the grass-roots and national levels. Organizations like the National Prostate Cancer Coalition, out of Washington, D.C., and the American Prostate Society, based in Maryland, are dedicated to informing the public about the dangers of prostate cancer and the importance of annual screening. Celebrities like golf great Arnold Palmer and former Temptations

131

singer Damon Harris have joined forces with Prostate Action Incorporated in helping men to make informed decisions about their prostate health.

Prostate cancer strikes one man in eight. But it is a slowly growing type of cancer and usually occurs in men over 60. Most males don't take the danger seriously, doctors say.

Anything having to do with elimination or reproduction causes squeamishness in many Americans—most of whom are also taught to "be a man" and "tough it out" when faced with pain or illness.

When they first consider the standard medical options, it's no wonder so many newly diagnosed men retreat into denial. The prostate's complicated location, amid a tangle of nerve bundles and muscle groups, makes it notoriously difficult to operate on or treat with radiation without damaging surrounding tissue. Resulting impotence and incontinence may be "a fate worse than death" to some men.

As medical ethician Arthur Caplan told *Newsweek*, "There isn't a right answer [to prostate cancer patients]. You can choose to have the surgery, if what matters to you is long life and you don't care if you become impotent or have a harder time peeing. Or someone at age 70 might decide, 'I'm not buying enough time to put those functions at risk."

Early prostate-cancer symptoms are identical to those of BPH and prostatitis, so most doctors will run routine blood and urine tests on any prostate patient to ensure that cancer cells aren't present. There is still some controversy over how widespread early detection tests should become and who should pay for them. But instead of arguing public policy, I will discuss the disease itself.

What Is Prostate Cancer?

Experts haven't yet discovered what causes prostate cancer, but they have connected it to high levels of the hormones testosterone and estradiol. They suspect that high-fat diets may stimulate production of these hormones.

Other links have been found in patients' heredity, sexual practices, past histoies of illness, injuries, and surgeries. (One study found that men who'd undergone vasectomies sometimes had a higher incidence of prostate cancer later.)

Cancer is basically a case of the body's own cells' having gone awry. When normal cells' growth processes are affected over time by *carcinogens*—cancer causing agents—they sometimes "mutate into cancer cells. These maverick cells grow more rapidly than usual and "take over" neighboring cells' growth apparatus. A cancer that starts in a particular organ frequently changes the blood chemistry or secretions of the organ, giving doctors a chemical warning sign.

About 40,000 men die a year after cancer cells in their prostates migrate—or *metastasize*—to their bones, lungs, or other organs.

With early detection and diagnosis, 90 percent of prostate-cancer patients live at least five years beyond their diagnosis and almost two-thirds live 10 years or more. Prostate cancer kills if not treated on time, however. Early detection is therefore of great importance.

Prostate cancer is the second-most deadly cancer among American men, just behind lung cancer. Health care experts estimate that if all 20 million at-risk American men were tested for prostate cancer, 400,000 would be found eligible for treatment. For now, about 180,000 new cases are diagnosed each year.

Prostate cancer usually grows very slowly and frequently stays right where it is instead of spreading through the body. Many men have prostate cancer for years and never know it—many cancers are found only after BPH treatments provide sample tissues. Postmortem exams frequently find undiagnosed prostate cancer in bodies that expired from an unrelated illness.

In other instances, however, doctors do find cancer, usually through a rectal exam. This 10-minute procedure is recommended by the American Cancer Society, which says every man over 40 should include one in his annual checkup. Doctors sometimes use an instrument called a *sigmoidoscope* to view the interior of the colon, where they look for internal cysts, hemorrhoids, or

DIGITAL EXAMINATION FOR PROSTATE CANCER

Pschyrembel Klinisches Worterbuch. DeGruyter, Berlin, Germany. 1986.

abnormal tissue.

Others settle for the rubber-glove approach; many men find a *digital examination* more comfortable, if not as comprehensive.

Those at risk for cancer can undergo a blood test that detects abnormal amounts of *prostatic specific antigen (PSA)*, a cancer indicator. (Critics point out that three out of four men will be the victims of false-positive readings with this test.) Dr. Isadore Rosenfeld describes these tests in his recent book *The Best Treatment*; he says that abnormally high PSA readings usually

PROSTATIC ASPIRATION TO DETERMINE THE PRESENCE OR ABSENCE OF PROSTATIC CANCER

Pschyrembel Klinisches Worterbuch. DeGruyter, Berlin, Germany. 1986.

prompt an *acid phosphatase test*, which tells if prostate cancer has metastasized to the bones.

Other routine diagnostic tools include *fine needle aspiration*, or a *needle biopsy*—the removal of a bit of the prostate tissue through an anally administered needle.

If a final diagnosis isn't obtained through this outpatient procedure, the doctor may schedule an ultrasound-guided laparascopic exam, similar to the TURP apparatus used to surgically reduce prostatic hypertrophy. (Rosenfeld calls this a "biopsy gun.") This secures bits of prostate tissue that should be sufficient for a diagnosis, and it can sometimes be done in a urologist's office.

If the diagnosis is cancer, several options can be considered. If the cancer is still limited to the prostate gland, there are still several choices, each with its avid advocates.

1. Watchful Waiting is the best option for those who are elderly, are uninsured, are in poor health, or have cancer samples that are "well-differentiated," or somewhat stable. Your doctor will want you to return to his office every three or four months for rectal exams and PSA tests. If and when the cancer begins to spread, more aggressive action can be taken. Those opposed to this approach, such as *Newsweek* magazine health writer Jerry Adler, say this "amounts to monitoring the tumor in expectation that something else will kill the patient first."

2. Radiation is another cancer-treatment option with its share of advocates and nay sayers. Dr. Rosenfeld writes that his patients find their long-term outlook is better with radiation than with "watchful waiting" as many as 85 percent live at least 10 more years following radiation. "Seeding" a tumor with radioactive pellets the size of rice grains is a popular treatment. It is less invasive and expensive than surgery, but it requires expert handling. Troublesome side effects include chronic diarrhea, exhaustion, rectal pain and fissures, incontinence, infections, and impotence.

3. Radical Prostatectomy, or surgical removal of the prostate through an abdominal incision, gives about the same chance for cure as radiation. It is the treatment of choice of American urologists: One survey said 80 percent of these doctors would recommend the surgery to a man in his 60s whose cancer was confined to the gland. In England, however, only 4 percent of the urologists said they would recommend the surgery; 92 percent of American radiation oncologists said they would advise against it.

Prostatectomy is a serious abdominal operation. It is risky, expensive, and of questionable value to men over 70 years old, according to a Dartmouth University study. Eight percent of men studied over age 75 suffered serious complications after the surgery; 2 percent died of them.

Radical Prostatectomy leaves up to 85 percent of patients impotent; 27 percent of patients are at least partially incontinent. Newer "nerve-sparing" surgical techniques are improving the odds for men concerned about sexual vigor, however and researchers say that less invasive surgical techniques are in the works.

The Dartmouth team told *Newsweek* that "if the medical community were to apply the same standards of safety and efficacy required for approval of new drugs ... it is likely that neither *radical prostatectomy* nor *radiation therapy* would be approved."

Even though thousands of men are treated with surgeries that have few scientific studies to back themup, the news is not all bad. Just look at Bob Dole, the former Republican leader of the U.S. Senate. His prostate was removed in 1991, but his aggressive energy is the bane of Democrats everywhere.

Cryosurgery is the newest wave in prostate-cancer treatment. With the patient under general anesthesia, doctors insert five metal probes between the scrotum and anus, eliminating the need for a deep incision. After placing the probes about the prostate with help from ultrasound imaging, the doctor then injects super-cooled nitrogen into the cancerous tissues. A computer monitors tissue destruction through the ultrasound system. After the surgery, the patient is left with several tiny incisions that the surgeon stitches closed. A urinary catheter will be placed in the bladder typically for one to two weeks following the surgery. The procedure requires only one or two nights in the hospital and causes little or no bleeding. Recovery is quick, and sexual potency is frequently spared.

Laser Surgery, which was discussed in Chapter 2 as a treatment for BPH, is still experimental in *prostate-cancer* cases, but some doctors see it as the surgery of choice for the future. Currently, it is used as an alternative to TURP or *radical prostatectomy* as a way to eliminate the cancerous gland altogether without opening the abdomen. Laser surgery is easy on the patient. It causes no bleeding or long recovery time, can be used with little or no anesthetic, can be repeated without ill effects, and is virtually painless.

Testosterone, a male hormone produced in the testicles, effectively "feeds" prostate cancer, researchers have found. Many men have the problem removed at its source, by having their testes surgically removed in an operation known as "orchiectomy." It is the oldest form of hormone treatment for *prostate cancer* and is frequently used to treat *testicular cancer* as well.

Rosenfeld recommends this surgical castration, even though he admits it sounds brutal. The operation can be done in a day, and small plastic balls are inserted into the scrotal sac for appearance's sake. This inevitably ends in impotence, however.

Nonsurgical Options

Hormone therapies are as popular as surgeries but are dismissed by many urologists as unproven. Many patients whose cancer has metastasized find relief through reducing the amount of male hormone in the bloodstream—the substance the cancer "feeds on." Without testosterone, impotency is almost inevitable.

One such drug is *diethyistibestrol (DES)*, a chemical similar to estrogen, a female hormone. Although DES brings with it a longer life and lessened symptoms, it isn't without side effects. It kills a man's sex drive, and many men report feminizing effects: breast enlargement, thinning beards, and scrotal shrinkage.

LH-RH Agonists (Leuprolide and Goserelin) can be used to treat even later stages of prostate cancer. This synthetic pituitary hormone therapy regulates the release of *testosterone* into the bloodstream. After triggering an initial rush of *testosterone*, it causes a drastic *decrease* in *testosterone*, which "starves" the tumor. Its only remarkable side effects are occasional hot flashes, headaches, or impotence. The agonists are usually administered through injections or implanted pellets.

LH-RH's inevitable downside is its longevity—effectiveness sometimes decreases after two years. It also affects only the pituitary gland, not the testosterone-producing cells in the testes. The small amount produced "down there" may be enough to keep a stray cancer cell or two alive.

Antiandrogens are hormones that inhibit the action of testosterone on cancer cells. Marketed through the brand name *Flutamide*, antiandrogens are frequently used in concord with other hormone treatments to lessen the pain of advanced prostate cancer.

Dr. Fernand LaBrie, a physician in the department of molecular endocrinology at Laval University Medical Center in Quebec, uses a "one-two punch" on his prostate-cancer patients. He combines a *Luprolide-type drug* with *Flutamide,* and he reports a 70 percent response rate to this therapy.

THE PROSTATE GLAND SHOWING THE DIFFERENT STAGES OF CANCER

STAGE T1 – Cancer is palpable on digital examination. It is small in size and is localized to one side of the prostate gland.

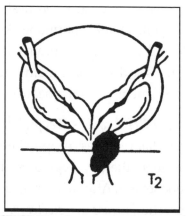

STAGE T2 – A more extensive form of cancer infiltration – detected through digital examination. Where it is thought that the cancer has not spread outside of the prostate gland.

STAGE T3 - Cancer is one in which the prostate cancer has spread outside the confines of the prostate gland. Detectable through digital examination.

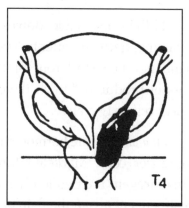

STAGE T4 – Cancer has spread outside the confines of the prostate gland and has metastasized.

Immunotherapy is a method used to build up the body's natural defenses against all diseases, including cancer. Some doctors combine *immunotherapy* with *chemotherapy* to help patients through later stages of prostate cancer. Other sufferers use natural cures and herbal soothers to help their bodies fight the cancer. Some of these are detailed in chapter 9.

Medical Investigational Treatments

Some doctors are seeing successful results from several new prostate-cancer treatments—used alone or in combination with other treatment options. Be aware that these methods are used only on an experimental basis, and it can take up to 15 years for scientists to prove the long-term effectiveness of any experimental option. Your doctor can inform you on where and what clinical trials are ongoing in your region. Ask him to contact the National Cancer Institute's Physicians' Direct Query, or "PDQ," referral system.

Radiation and "Hyperthermia"

Scientists know that temperatures of 105 degrees F or above are deadly to cell division and weak cells. They are attempting to put this information to work on prostate cancer by combining it with radiation to kill cancer cells.

Dr. Isaac Kaver of the University of Virginia wrote in the medical journal *Urology* that heat makes cancer cells more sensitive to radiation. Application of heat to the whole body or to the localized tumor area prior to radiation was more effective at killing the cells than using either treatment alone, Kaver wrote.

High-energy Radiation

Another variation on standard radiation therapy is *high linear energy transfer radiation.* Instead of using the usual X-ray or gamma-ray radiation, this method employs "accelerators" that use helium ions, neutrons, and protons to penetrate to deep-seated tumors and irradiate the cancer tissues. Some experts say this is more effective than standard radiation therapy. It is available, however, at only a few sites throughout the continent.

In hyperthermia treatment of the prostate, a microwave probe is placed through the urethra into the prostate and the prostate is heated to 105 degrees F. Some of the prostatic tissues are destroyed, and the gland shrinks. The gland is also reported to be softer after treatment, allowing for easier urination. While not widely used, this technique did receive FDA approval in 1995.

Enzyme-inhibiting Drugs are already in use for treatment of benign prostatic hypertrophy. *Finasteride (Proscar),* a drug discussed in chapter 3, is also being studied as an early-stage cancer treatment. *Finasteride* works by blocking production of an enzyme that triggers production of a testosterone byproduct that "feeds" prostate tumors. *Suramin,* a drug with exotic origins, is also being studied. Originally used to treat African sleeping sickness, it may, some researchers are finding, interfere with tumor growth.

Chemotherapy is usually considered a last resort for cancer patients. It uses chemicals to directly attack cancer cells but usually ends up killing many healthy cells as well. However, an experimental group of 25 men written up in *Urology* showed a significant (50 percent) drop in PSA levels after being treated with a combination of standard chemotherapy drugs.

Biological Therapy

Like the immunotherapy option listed above, this experimental method involves the use of substances meant to trigger the body's natural defenses against disease.

Colony-stimulating factors are produced within the body and trigger production of white blood cells—the body's protectors against disease. Scientists say use of colony-stimulators allows higher doses of chemotherapy to be used to target the cancer directly.

T-Cells recognize and attack cancer cells. Scientists are experimenting with removing *T-cells* from the blood, fortifying them, boosting their reproduction, and then returning them to the body to attack the cancer. *Tumor necrosis factors* are tumor-destroying proteins. Scientists are trying to find a way to trigger increased production of these proteins within the body.

Other researchers are working on "designer proteins" called *monoclonal antibodies*. These natural cancer-attackers go after specific types of cancer. Doctors hope to someday attach medication or radiation to these proteins to better deliver relief to the affected organs and tissues.

Interleukins and *interferons* are proteins the body makes to fight off infections. Scientists are studying the effects these proteins can have against cancer.

Interleukin-2 (IL-2) stimulates the body's white blood cells', ability to destroy cancer. In fact doctors can remove white blood cells from a cancer patient, mix them with IL-2, and return them to the patient's bloodstream to help fight the cancer.

Early studies of this therapy have shown it to be effective in shrinking certain solid tumors. The therapy is, however, far from 100 percent effective and comes with serious side effects, including fluid retention that could lead to organ failure.

IL-2 therapy has already been approved by the FDA to treat metastasized kidney and melanoma cancers. Scientists are now researching the effectiveness of *IL-2 therapy* against other cancers, including the colorectal, ovarian, lung, brain, breast, and prostate varieties.

Interferons are natural cancer-fighting proteins found in the body. Studies have shown that interferons can improve the immune systems of cancer patients. By slowing down a cancer cell's growth, interferons may force it to act more like a normal cell. A promising 50 percent reduction in tumor size has been documented in some patients, and leukemia patients have responded well to the therapy over half the time.

The FDA has approved interferon therapy to treat certain cancers, including leukemia and Kaposi's sarcoma. Further studies are being conducted to find out if the therapy could be effective for other types of cancer.

Oncogene therapy is a genetic approach to cancer treatment. Scientists have discovered that normal genes—the tiny protein chains that carry a cell's genetic information—can sometimes, somehow, change into cancer-promoting genes called *oncogenes*.

An upbeat accompaniment was the discovery of *suppressor genes*—a concurrent group of genes that sometimes forestall production of oncogenes. As detailed in Shapiro's *Prostate Problems*, the discovery opens up a new realm of treatment possibilities— *"gene therapy"* for cancer-prone patients. Doctors may someday replace oncogenes or faulty suppressor genes with "good" genes.

Metastasis: Stopping the Spread

Scientists at the National Cancer Institute have recently found several new clues as to why cancer spreads and are working on therapies that could stop cancer where it starts. A piece in the

Scientific American detailed the breakthroughs.

In order for a cancer cell to spread, it has to detach from its original location and hitch a ride through a blood or lymph vessel to a new location where it can start a new cellular base. The body has a number of controls that keep normal cells in place, and the cancerous cell must avoid these controls in order to survive. A cell cannot normally detach from its site and survive a trip to another location. If a healthy cell becomes unattached, a signal is sent to the cell that indicates its status and the cell responds by stopping its own growth and dying.

Scientists are unsure exactly how cancer cells manage to avoid cell death when they metastasize, but they suspect that ocogenes, mutated versions of normal genes, give a false signal to the nucleus of the cancer cell that it's properly attached when in fact it isn't. Having been fooled by this false signal, the cancer cell does not stop growing and die as a normal cell would.

Metalloproteinases, enzymes secreted by cancer cells, were linked to metastasis by several researchers. They are working on ways to inhibit production or change the composition of these enzymes, which break down the defensive cell walls of healthy tissues and allow cancer cells to invade.

Caring for Your Testicles

Other threats men face from "down there" are orchitis, or *inflammation of the testes*, and *cancer of the testes*.

Orchitis can strike younger men as well as the middle-aged and elderly, and it is frequently "let go to pass on its own" by men too embarrassed to consult a doctor. Unfortunately, overlooking a case of orchitis could result in later infertility.

Orchitis, like *prostatitis*, is frequently caused by a bacterial infection inside the organs—not necessarily venereal disease. Orchitis can indicate tuberculosis or mumps infections elsewhere

CROSS-SECTION OF MALE GENITOURINARY TRACT

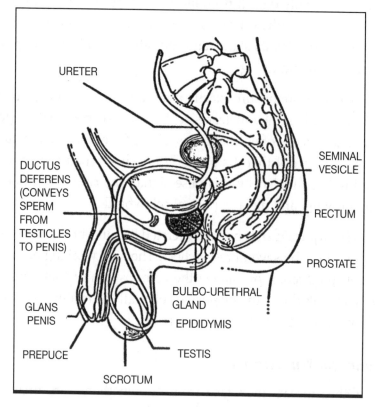

in the body.

Folk medicine has found several cures and pain relievers for noncancerous *orchitis*. The plant extract from *Echinacea* is especially effective against *testicular swelling*. Ten to 20 drops, taken hourly through the day, work well with nighttime mudpacks to bring down swelling and take away pain. To keep the mud paste from drying out, add a tablespoon of *Saint-John's-wort oil* to the paste or use a compress made from *squeezed cabbage leaves*. (If this causes a strong skin reaction, remove it immediately.)

Testicular cancer isn't very common, but it is most likely to strike men between the ages of 18 and 32 and in those over 60. Scientists have linked this to the thymus gland, which is very active in young men and suddenly becomes inactive at about age 60.

THE SPREAD OF TESTICULAR CANCER

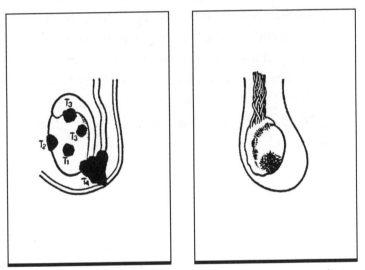

These two pictures show the eventual spread of testicular cancer if it is left unchecked. A quick, monthly self-examination can help a man to detect this cancer in its early stages when it can be successfully treated. The shaded areas show where the cancer most likely can manifest itself.

Left untreated, *testicular cancer* can lead to death. When, however, it is detected early, it is 100 percent curable, doctors say.

Every man needs to know how to perform a simple monthly self-examination for testicular cancer. The exam is easy, quick, and very effective—and it could save your life.

INSTRUCTIONS

A SELF-EXAMINATION FOR TESTICULAR CANCER

Hold the testicles with both hands, being careful not to let them slip. Massage gently the entire surface of the testicles, checking for any hard lumps. Make sure you don't mistake the epididymis for a harmful growth—it is a soft, sausage-shaped "bump" that runs down the back of the testicles. The "wiry" texture within the scrotum is normal, too—it simply carries the sperm away from the testes. Should you feel any "knots," "pebbles," or "peas" or notice unusual puckers or "dents" in the skin, contact your doctor immediately.

· CHAPTER 9 ·

Natural Help for Prostate Cancer

Even with all the research and experiments going on, the average man with prostate cancer may want more options to choose from. There are unproven "cures" and plenty of "quacks" ready to prey on gullible or desperate cancer patients, but careful research will reveal that doctors and hospitals aren't the only places where at least relief can be found if not a cure.

Even men who have no *prostate symptoms*—or a simple case of *prostatitis*—can benefit from many of the natural therapies outlined here. After all, today's healthy prostate may well fall prey to cancer as it ages. And as mothers say the world over, "An ounce of prevention is worth a pound of cure."

So even if it's too late for *prostate-cancer* prevention, putting common sense precautions into use could save you from developing cancer elsewhere in your body. Cut back on your alcohol intake, limit your exposure to the sun, stop smoking and avoid inhaling other smokers' fumes, start an exercise program, get regular check-ups, and perform recommended self-examinations for mysterious lumps. Also, avoid environmental hazards like chemical fumes, dust, and industrial pollutants.

It is also important to note that many "natural cures," thought in the past to be part of simple folklore, have been proven through laboratory tests to be directly beneficial to patients. Many medical doctors now prescribe treatments similar to those their grandparents used.

As I stated before, diet is the key to cancer treatment and prevention. Altering your intake of certain substances may work much like the immunotherapies prescribed by doctors—they build up the body's natural cancer defenses, or interfere with the chemical processes that cause cancer to spread.

Fiber and Prostate Cancer: The Seventh-day Adventist Study

Researchers at California's Loma Linda School of Medicine studied the diets and health of "normal" men as opposed to men who are observant memebers of the Seventh-day Adventist church, which prescribes a vegetarian diet. The researchers found that the Adventists—who eat twice the amount of dietary fiber as the average men—had a markedly lower incidence of *prostate cancer*. The researchers concluded that the vegetarians' low-fat and high-fiber diets help rid their bodies of excess hormone secretions, thus lowering their chances of developing prostate difficulties.

The study created a flurry of "high-fiber" diets and programs until another study disproved some of its more extravagant claims. But a wise male will be sure to consume plenty of fresh vegetables and whole grains—thousands of healthy Adventist prostates can't be wrong!

Fruits, vegetables, berries, figs, and dates are good sources of fiber, as are brans and whole grains.

Tomatoes and Lycopene

One exciting new development in the fight against prostate cancer can be found right in the produce department of your local grocery store. The simple tomato has received praise for the powerful punch it packs against prostate cancer. Tomatoes contain a potent antioxidant called lycopene. Like other antioxidants, it neutralizes harmful substances in the body that are felt to contribute to causing cancer.

Studies show a connection between eating tomato products and reducing the risk of developing prostate cancer. One large, five-year, study found an incredible one-third drop in the risk of developing prostate cancer for men who ate 10 servings a week of cooked tomatoes as compared to those that ate less than two servings. Another telling study, headed by Dr. Omer Kucuk, Professor of Medicine and Oncology at the Barbara Ann Karmanos Cancer Institute in Detroit, Michigan, followed 30 men with prostate cancer who were scheduled to have their prostates removed. Three weeks before their scheduled surgery, study participants were randomly given either 15-milligram lycopene supplements twice a day or nothing at all. The lycopene group saw their PSA levels drop 20 percent before their surgery, while the untreated group's PSA levels stayed the same. Perhaps the most surprising result of the study was that the tumors in those men who were given lycopene were actually starting to shrink prior to surgery and that the spread of their cancers was found to be 42 percent lower than those of the untreated group.

With the evidence building in the tomato's favor, an independent review of 72 separate studies searching for any possible links between the risk of developing prostate cancer and eating tomato products was conducted by Dr. Edward Giovannucci of Harvard Medical School. What Dr. Giovannucci found was that well over half of those studies did connect eating tomato products with a reduced risk.

Tomatoes are cheap and readily available, and eating them is a tasty way for you to fight off prostate cancer. Try adding at least 10 servings of tomatoes to your diet a week. Pasta with tomato sauce, pizza, soups, salsas, juice, canned tomatoes, ketchup, and salads with fresh tomatoes can all count toward your goal of 10 servings a week. Although fresh tomatoes are packed with lypocene, cooking the tomatoes, which breaks down the cell walls, makes it easier for your body to use the substance. Adding some monounsaturated fat, such as olive oil, when the tomatoes are cooked, will raise the amount of lypocene your body absorbs even more. Lycopene can also be found in smaller concentrations in watermelon, red grapefruit, and dried apricots.

Fatty Acids: Omega-3 and Omega-6

A vegetarian diet is by definition a low-fat diet, another element that may contribute to freedom from cancer. Some researchers have linked human cancers to animal feed—almost all cattle, hogs, and chickens raised for human consumption are fed artificial animal growth hormones to fatten them up and hasten their final trip to market.

Some researchers say these hormones remain in the meat and act in odd ways on humans who consume them. No one has directly linked the animal hormones to human cancer, but it is a theory worth considering. Some prostate patients—some of them beef farmers—will eat only "free-range" or kosher meat for this reason. In fact, European Union farmers have had a ban on giving hormones to cattle since 1988 because of health fears.

While a fat-laden diet may contribute to prostate cancer, it should not be confused with the body's need for essential fatty acids. Research discovered that *Omega-3*, a fatty acid abundant in fish oil, may be an effective cancer fighter as well as a noted element in the reduction of heart-attack risk.

Scientists studied the diets of people in Greenland, Iceland, Japan and China whose diets revolve around their abundant fisheries. Almost none of the people suffered from *breast* or *prostate cancer*. When the study focused on people from the same ethnic groups who live and eat "Western-style," cancer incidence rose to average levels.

A study at Rutgers University and the Memorial Sloan Kettering Cancer Center found that *fish-oil* supplements reduced the size, weight, and incidence of cancerous tumors in cancer-induced laboratory mice.

Humans are not mice. But ongoing studies support the *Omega-3* study and show beneficial effects at preventing cancer, if not helping alleviate its symptoms. The best available source of *Omega-3* is salmon. If availability or expense is an obstacle, try *salmon oil*—also available in capsule form at health-food stores.

Other essential fatty acids are associated with lessened prostate symptoms. *Linolenic acid* and *linoleic acid* (*Omega-3* and *Omega-6*), found in *flaxseed* and *pumpkin-seed oils*, are involved in the production of prostaglandins—chemicals associated with sexual vitality.

Pumpkin seeds are used with success by many men who suffer BPH symptoms, according to *Nutritional Research News*. It is thought the seeds' concentrations of zinc, magnesium, and phosphorus help decrease *prostate inflammation*.

Vitamin A: Hooray!

Researchers at the University of Arizona Cancer Center started another trend in 1982 when they announced they use Vitamin A as part of their anticancer arsenal.

Mark Bricklin describes their experiments in his *Encyclopedia of Natural Healing*: Mice injected with vitamin A responded remarkably better to radiation treatments than did mice without the injections. Mice treated with only vitamin A or only radiation survived about two months after therapy ceased. Those treated with combination therapy survived 10 months, with less than 10 percent showing tumor regrowth.

Since then, doctors have found positive links between intake of vitamin A and a lessened incidence of lung cancer in men. A comprehensive prostate-cancer study undertaken in Japan revealed a substantially lower death rate from prostate cancer among men who ate green and yellow vegetables each day. Japanese scientists theorized that its the carotene—vitamin A—in these vegetables that may be responsible.

Foods rich in carotene include carrots, sweet potatoes, squash, spinach, broccoli, pumpkins, kale, and sweet red peppers. Studies in Wisconsin and Scotland found that even those cancer patients in relatively good health whose vitamin A levels were lower than average did not respond as well to chemotherapy as patients whose diets were rich in carotene.

A landmark research study by the American Institute for Cancer Research (AICR) found that 60 percent to 70 percent of all incidences of cancer could be prevented through dietary factors. Diet is under the control of individuals—and changing engrained bad habits in regard to diet can drastically cut cancer risks.

F O O D S   R I C H   I N   V I T A M I N   A

5 oz. sweet potato	15,000 IU
2 to 3 apricots	15,000 IU
1 cup peas and carrots	15,000 IU
1 cup baked butternut squash	13,000 IU
1 raw carrot	5,000 IU
1/2 mango	4,800 IU
1/4 cantaloupe	3,500 IU
1 stalk broccoli	3,500 IU
1 raw tomato	1,800 IU
1/3 papaya	1,750 IU
1 cup asparagus	51,500 IU

IU = International Unit

The Vitamin E Connection

Taking a vitamin E supplement each day may be the key to keeping prostate troubles away. Vitamin E, another one of nature's powerful antioxidants, has already been shown to stimulate immune function, have positive cardiovascular effects, and potentially decrease the DNA damage that can eventually lead to cancer. Really conclusive evidence was lacking, however, until September 2000, when the University of Utah School of Medicine reported that Vitamin E significantly inhibits the growth of human prostate cells. Researchers in the Division of Nutrition at the University of Texas concurred with these findings. Their Vitamin E research confirmed that the vitamin does trigger cell death in human prostate-cancer cells without affecting the normal prostate cells. In other words, Vitamin E has been shown to not only stop the spread of prostate cancer cells but also to actually kill them. More research is needed, of course, but these findings are extremely exciting.

The U.S. recommended dietary allowance for adult men is 10 milligrams or 15 IUs, of Vitamin E daily. This dosage is probably too conservative. Most experts agree that a dosage of 400 IUs to 800 IUs a day should provide the protective effects you are seeking.

You can add more Vitamin E to your diet by choosing the right foods. Foods high in Vitamin E include almonds, sunflower seeds, wheat germ, broccoli, spinach, and fish.

Vitamin E is very safe for most people. However, taking more than 800 IUs a day is not advisable. If you are already on a blood-thinning medication, you should check with your doctor; very high doses of vitamin E (more than 1,800 IUs a day) could increase the effects of such drugs. As always, you should check with your physician regarding your individual situation before adding any supplements or vitamins to your diet.

Vitamin D, The Sunshine Vitamin

It has long been known that vitamin D, the sunshine vitamin, plays an important role in bone and mineral metabolism. During the Industrial Revolution, when child labor flourished children who did not get sufficient doses of sunlight daily suffered from stunted growth and abnormal development. Now, low blood levels of vitamin D have been found in prostate cancer patients. Recent studies have shown that vitamin D inhibits the growth of prostate-cancer cells and triggers their death. It appears to bind to the cancer cells and cause apoptosis, or a transformation into less malignant cells. These findings suggest that vitamin D may have potential as a cancer preventive.

Many turn to milk and other dairy products enriched with vitamin D for a primary source of this substance. However, studies have linked a high dietary intake of dairy and meat products to an increased risk of prostate cancer. Researchers theorize that higher calcium levels and/or phosphorous from dairy products may actually lower the circulating blood levels of vitamin D.

The current U.S. recommended dietary allowance (RDA) of vitamin D is 200 IUs. However, according to a review in the *American Journal of Clinical Nutrition* by Dr. Reinhold Vieth of the University of Toronto, adults should be getting a minimum of 1,000 IUs to obtain its cancer-fighting benefits. Vitamin D occurs naturally in small quantities in only a few foods, such as sardines, salmon, swordfish, and butter. The easiest, and most natural way, to add more Vitamin D to your diet is to spend some time in the sun every day.

Although a rare occurrence, large amounts of Vitamin D can potentially be toxic. Please check with your physician before taking more than the daily RDA and watch for side effects like headaches, nausea, dizziness, vomiting, loss of appetite, and dry mouth.

Carbohydrates and Fats

The National Cancer Institute advises Americans to keep their total fat intake to less than 30 percent of their diets and to increase their intake of complex carbohydrates.

So where should you begin? Start with fruits and vegetables. They are ideal sources of complex carbohydrates, as well as vitamins and minerals. Complex carbohydrates are a natural aid to dieters, as they produce a filled-up feeling without a huge calorie load. They are also a natural energy source.

Don't confuse complex carbohydrates with simple carbohy-drates—a man-made byproduct of refining and processing natural foods. Commercial white sugar, white bread, potato chips, and corn chips are good examples of how man takes an excellent product of nature and crushes, dyes, or fries it into a nutritional nightmare.

If you are fond of potatoes, eat baked ones topped with a little broccoli and melted mozzarella cheese. You'll be surprised at how filling a potato prepared in this way is, and it has less than 225 calories. Complex carbohydrates and fibers should be balanced with dairy products and protein for a balanced nutritional intake. It's not difficult to choose low-fat dairy products instead of their high-calorie counterparts. When choosing a protein source, choose lean cuts of meat, or, better yet, poultry, fish, beans, peas, or tofu.

By simply concentrating on eating lots of complex carbohydrates and fiber and fewer dairy products and proteins, you'll see the hid-den payoff—a diet that is lower overall in fat. You'll feel satisfied with fewer calories.

Cornell University researchers tested the effects of such a diet as opposed to those of high- and medium-fat diets.

People on the low-fat diet ate as much food as they wanted but consumed 627 fewer calories than their counterparts.

A Macrobiotics Diet for Prostate Cancer

Back in 1975, Mr. M. was diagnosed with prostate cancer. He was in his mid-50s.

Despite his undergoing conventional treatments under his doc-tor's direction, the cancer spread into his spine, hip, and shoulder.

Surgery was performed to remove a portion of one testicle, and radiation and chemotherapy were administered. Mr.M. also took hormone-therapy pills, but his outlook continued to dim. Chemotherapy was particularly hard for him. His pain continued, and he vomited for up to 12 hours after each treatment

By 1980, he'd had enough of chemotherapy. He agreed to continue the hormone treatments, though—and consulted with a doctor who recommended he try a macrobiotic diet.

Mr.M. noticed results almost immediately. His appetite and energy returned. In a month's time, he was able to cut his hormone consumption in half, and after six months, his doctor discontinued it altogether—the pain was gone.

M. knew intuitively, by the way his body felt, that he was well along the way of conquering his prostate cancer. He decided to confirm this feeling by having a bone scan done—an X-ray view of his skeleton. M. and his doctor both did a double take when the films came back. The malignancy had shrunk considerably. The shoulder, spine, and hip were clear of the dark shadows of cancer that had previously appeared there.

As you may imagine, M. became an enthusiastic supporter of the macrobiotic way of life. "I am totally convinced that we are what we eat and that we literally destroy our bodies with the poor-quality foods we consume. I take in a reasonable amount of exercise and look on cancer as something we can overcome with diet and determination," M. explained. "We have amazing bodies. They can heal themselves if we furnish them with the proper nourishment and eliminate the harmful variety."

M.'s healing discovery comes from the Orient, where human culture traditionally lives in harmony with nature. Macrobiotics is a method of extending life and conquering disease—including cancer—by consuming food derived from one's immediate environment.

Before the days of refrigerated shipping and worldwide food imports and exports, everybody followed a macrobiotic diet. Those who lived on the plains of Africa and America ate plenty of grains and fruits along with an occasional serving of wild meat. Eskimos consumed fish and high-fat preserved meats, which helped them conserve body heat. Each society followed a diet very different from the others, but they all provided the nutrients their environments demanded for human survival.

Chinese, Korean, and Japanese groups adopted and adapted the macrobiotic diets of their ancestors and passed the dietary practices on to their children.

In more recent years, Micho Kushi, a Chinese nutrition consultant, refined the ancient macrobiotic concept to match the needs of modern Americans. His diet is designed to provide a perfect balance of nutrients required by healthy cells. These foods assist the body's natural elimination of built-up toxins, fats, and mucus—all of which clog the tissues and cells and lead to disease.

The standard macrobiotic diet is heavy on whole grains, beans, and cooked vegetables, along with certain supplementary foods, drinks and Oriental condiments. Ideally, most of the vegetable and grain items should be grown within 50 miles of your home—the very best are those grown in your backyard garden!

Fifty percent to 60 percent of each meal should be *whole* grains: *brown rice, oats, corn, barley, buckwheat,* and *millet.* Another 25 percent to 30 percent should be fresh vegetables like *cabbage, carrots, turnips (with their tops), onions, squash, cauliflower, Swiss chard, bok choy, watercress, burdock root,* and other locally grown produce.

Eat up to a third of your vegetables raw, in salads. Kushi warns, however, that those suffering from cancer should be careful to limit their intake of raw foods, and should cook their vegetables before eating.

Vegetables high in acid or fat should be excluded from a macrobiotic diet. They include *tomatoes, eggplant, potatoes, asparagus, spinach, yams, beets, zucchini, avocados,* and *peppers.*

Beans and sea vegetables are important parts of macrobiotics, too. Recommended low-fat beans include *lentils, chickpeas, and azuki beans.* Mineral-rich sea vegetables like *hiziki, kombu, wakame, nori, seaweed,* and *Irish moss* are available at health-food stores or Oriental markets. They can be eaten as a side dish or added to soup.

Soup consumption, however, should be limited to two small bowls per day. It should be prepared with recommended beans, vegetables, or whole grains and should always include some wakame seaweed, experts say.

The diet allows drinks like cereal-grain coffees; spring water drunk at room temperature; teas made from roasted barley, brown rice, or bancha twigs; and dandelion tea.

This is only a small taste of the macrobiotics diet. Some say its wondrous effects are due to the trained specialists who tailor each diet to the needs of the patient. These dietitians are available at local chapters of the Kushi Institute, which supplies referrals, nutrition counseling, cooking classes, and courses on macrobiotic philosophy. For more information write it's national headquarters:

The Kushi Institute

P.O. Box 7

Becket, MA 01223

(413)623-5742

Simply Soy

The simple soybean is a powerful prostate-cancer fighter. Scientists have speculated for some time that isoflavones, plant-derived nutrients that are more concentrated in soy than in other plant-based foods, have the ability to ward off cancer. Now they have some evidence to back up that theory. One soy-derived isoflavon, genistein, has been proven to actually suppress human prostate-cancer cells. AntiCancer Inc., out of San Diego, California, has concluded a study showing that the growth of both human BPH tissue and prostate-cancer tissue is diminished when treated with just 1.25-10 micrograms of genistein.

Statistics show that Asian men, who eat a traditional diet high in soy-derived products and low in fat and calories, have a very low incidence of prostate cancer. In the United States, however, prostate cancer is the most commonly diagnosed form of non-skin cancer affecting men, with about 180,000 new cases diagnosed a year. Current evidence indicates that diet plays a significant role in the development and progression of prostate cancer. In fact, researchers found that as early as 1975 prostate-cancer deaths in 32 countries were linked to high-fat, Western-influenced diets. One Stanford University School of Medicine study dramatically demonstrated this effect when researchers concluded that Asian men who migrate from the Far East to the United States have their risk of prostate cancer double.

Asian men typically eat up to 10 times the amount of isoflavone-packed soy products a day as American men do. Japanese men consume up to 200 milligrams of soy-based isoflavones a day, followed by other Asian men who take in 25 to 45 milligrams a day. In stark contrast, the typical American man consumes less than 5 milligrams.

In addition to being a powerful prostate-cancer fighter, soy is also a good source of fiber, B vitamins, calcium, and Omega-3 essential fatty acids. The Food and Drug Administration (FDA) now recognizes soy's heart-healthy benefits and recommends that adults add 25 grams of soy protein to their daily diet. Soy has even been shown to lower total blood cholesterol and decrease so called "bad" cholesterol, or LDL.

With all of the positive publicity soy has been getting recently, it's easier now to incorporate it into your diet. In fact, you no longer have to make a special trip to a health-food store. Neighborhood grocery stores are keeping their shelves stocked with various soy products. You can get tofu, a soft cheese-like soy product, in a variety of tasty flavors. Try adding some lemon pepper tofu to your steamed veggies or cooking some sun-dried tomato and basil flavor to toss into your salads. Substitute a slice of soy cheese for your regular slice of American cheese on your broccoli or toast. You can substitute some soy flour for part of the regular white flour in pancakes, muffins, breads, or cakes. Roasted soy nuts, with a consistency resembling peanuts, are a delicious crunchy snack.

A concern about soy and a possible link to cognitive decline did surface after a study published in the *Journal of the American College of Nutrition* announced a possible link between eating large amounts of tofu (two or more servings a week) and a decline in mental health in later life. The longitudinal study began in 1965 to examine heart disease, stroke, and cancer in a group of Japanese-American men in Hawaii. Both the article presenting the study and an accompanying editorial made it clear that those men who ate the most tofu had a number of other factors that could have contributed to their mental deterioration for example, they were older, they had spent more years in Japan in poverty, and they had higher incidences of stroke. There is no conclusive evidence that tofu caused the effect researchers observed. The limited information on the participants' diets, along with the fact that there are no supporting follow-up studies, has caused many experts to doubt any conclusions concerning a link between soy and cognitive decline.

An Austrian "Naturopathic" Treatment for Prostate Malignancy

The Austrians look to herbs to help them deal with prostate cancer. Several of the herb-tea recipes provided in previous chapters will give prostate-cancer patients needed relief of symptoms while medical treatments are tried

Please note that these diets are not meant to treat or cure cancer or any other prostate complaint—they are supplements to a doctor's care, NOT substitutes for it.

The Austrian naturopath *Rudolph Breuss*, who created the treatment below, is credited with preventing and even curing a wide range of cancers, including *prostate cancer*.

He, too, testified to the effectiveness of the *small-flower-willow herb*. Patients should sip two cups of cold tea each day, made by simmering a pinch of willow herb in a pint of hot water.

He also suggested a *three-week regimen* of "kidney tea," an herbal mixture that cleanses and soothes the urinary tract.

Kidney tea is only part of this doctor's "total cure for cancer." His philosophy holds that a cancer tumor is an autonomous growth and can only be eliminated by a speical 42-day fast combined with a juice and tea therapy. Although the regimen is rigorous, most patients don't lose much weight. Recipes for two other important herbal teas in this treatment are given later.

• INSTRUCTIONS •

KIDNEY TEA – THREE WEEKS' SUPPLY

Mix together the following:

15 grams horsetail

10 grams nettle (best picked in spring)

8 grams birdknot grass

6 grams Saint-John's-wort

To Brew: Place a pinch of the mixture in a cup of almost-boiling water. Allow to steep for 10 minutes and then strain. Add 2 cups of hot water and boil for 10 minutes; then strain again.

To use: Drink a half-cup of this tea, cold,as the first thing you do in the morning, before lunch. and again before bed. **Take for three weeks only**. Wait another two or three weeks and, then resume. Do not eat meat broth, beef, or pork while on this regimen. Normal urination should resume after three days of starting the kidney-tea regimen.

• INSTRUCTIONS •

SAGE TEA

Place 1 or 2 teaspoons of sage in a pint of water and boil for three minutes. Add a pinch of Saint John's-wort, lemon balm, and peppermint. Steep for 10 minutes and then strain.

CRANESBILL TEA (GERANIUM ROBERTIANUM)

Cut very fine a large stem of Geranium robertianum, enough to make one full tablespoon. Add to 1 cup of very hot water and steep for 10 minutes.

Drink cold. Do not add sugar to either tea.*

The 42-day cancer treatment limits patients to recommended teas and a special vegetable juice. The juice satisfies hunger pangs, but patients should be careful to drink no more than a pint per day of the vegetable mixture. **The juice must be taken by the spoonful, slowly, so it mixes with saliva before it is swallowed.**

• INSTRUCTIONS •

VEGETABLE JUICE MIXTURE

Combine in a juicer or food processor all of the following:

3 parts red beets

1 part carrots

1 part celery

1 small radish

1 egg-size potato

Use a juicer to liquefy the vegetables.

NOTE: If the potato taste spoils the mixture for you, you can omit it here and instead drink a cup of potato peel tea each day. Put a handful of potato peelings in a pint of water and boil for two to four minutes.

* IMPORTANT: DO NOT use any form of sugar
during this 42-day fast for cancer treatment in
teas, or elsewhere.

SUGGESTED DIET ROUTINE

Upon waking:	one-half cup of cold kidney tea, sipped slowly
An hour later:	one or two cups of sage tea
An hour after that:	a small mouthful of vegetable juice
Half an hour later:	a small mouthful of vegetable juice
Lunchtime:	10-15 mouthfuls of vegetable juice
	Sage tea, unsugared
	One-half cup of cold kidney tea
Afternoon:	Mouthfuls of vegetable juice as needed
	Sage tea, unsugared
	One cup cranesbill tea
	One-half cup cold kidney tea

After the 42-day regimen ends, slowly begin to eat light solid food again—but nothing heavily salted. Continue to drink about half a cup of vegetable juice each day before meals for two to four weeks. Augment the treatment with light exercise and plenty of fresh air.

Naturopaths believe this cancer "cure" will not work on smokers who continue their habit.

Those coping with a *prostate-cancer* problem will do well to review the herbal relievers listed in chapter 5. Whether the swelling and pain rises from *cancer*, BPH, or *prostatitis symptoms*, herbs like the *small-flower willow* and *damiana* are proven to provide welcome relief.

Green Tea

The Chinese have been using green tea medicinally for centuries. Asian countries like China and Japan have long regarded it as a cancer fighter. In these countries, where prostate-cancer rates are much lower than in the United States, the average person drinks up to 10 cups of green tea a day. With so much anecdotal evidence available, researches have finally taken a more in-depth look at green tea, as Western science finally begins to catch up with Eastern medicine.

Polyphenols, antioxidants found in all plants, are naturally high in tea. Scientists from the Mayo Clinic uncovered a compound in the polyphenols of green tea, called epigalllocatechin-3-gallate, or ECGC, that inhibits human prostate-cancer cell growth and kills the cancerous cells. Researchers at Case Western University recently confirmed the effectiveness of ECGC in causing apoptosis, or cell death of human prostate-cancer cells, with their study published in April of 2000

While it's too early to state that green tea can prevent prostate cancer in humans, or even definitely slow its progress, the evidence clearly points in that direction. With increasing interest in its cancer-fighting abilities, green tea has become readily available in most local grocery stores.

Saw Palmetto

In an earlier chapter, I spoke of the saw palmetto's power to reduce the troublesome symptoms of BPH. Researchers are now concentrating on the cancer-fighting abilities of the extract. A team lead by Dr. C. Pail Sharma of Boston Bioproducts Inc. wanted to find out if the berry has any effect on prostate cancer cells. Team members set up a laboratory experiment in which they exposed both prostate-cancer cells and generic cancer cells to different amounts of the saw palmetto extract. They found that saw palmetto did, in fact, slow the growth of the cancerous prostate cells. A follow-up study by this same team found that a protein known as Cox-2, which has been linked to increased incidences of prostate cancer, was reduced in all cancer cells treated with saw palmetto. Although the researchers stress that their research is in its early stages, they concluded that there is enough evidence to warrant a man's taking a supplement containing saw palmetto extract.

When looking to add saw palmetto to your routine, make sure to read the labels to find one indicating that the preperation is an extract and not crushed whole berries. A dose of 160 milligrams twice a day is recommended.

A Natural Alternative to Constipation

One simple way to relieve prostate-cancer pain—or simply the pain of a swollen gland—is to keep your bowels clear. Constipation can add to the abdominal congestion caused by bladder and prostate complaints, making a bad situation downright miserable.

Constipation is defined as "the abnormally delayed or infrequent passage of dry, hardened feces." It is important to understand that a bowel movement is not necessarily "abnormally delayed" if one doesn't occur naturally every day. Every body is different; some people need to "go" once or twice daily, whereas others only evacuate their bowels every other day or so. When the digestive tract is functioning properly, the body maintains its own rhythm and doesn't require a stimulant laxative.

Sadly, the discomfort, embarrassment and pain of constipation symptoms are a way of life for many. Long-term constipation has been linked to maladies like *varicose veins, hemorrhoids, and* even *high blood pressure.*

Aside from organic causes like *spastic bowel syndrome, tumors,* and *diverticulitis,* much constipation occurs because of bad bowel habits. Normal intestinal functioning demands that we allow the bowels to move when they will—a lower intestine can fill up in less than six hours. However, through habit, many have trained their bodies to retain waste for 24 hours or more. When nature calls, the urge should be answered quickly—to avoid developing bad bowel habits that may lead to constipation.

The German *Handbuch fur Manner mit Prostataleiden* ("Handbook for Men With Prostate Problems") says constipation worsens cooperative functions of the bladder and its emptying muscle. When you are constipated, the increased volume of your bowels puts pressure on the pelvic organs. Common cholesterol buildup adds even more pressure to the stressed region. Symptoms like shivers and chills sometimes result—a condition the German text calls "cold constriction." The bladder muscle tightens up because of the body-wide chill and thus constricts urine flow.

Bladder and bowel complaints also result from too much heat. Upholstered furniture, too many sweaters, and overheated rooms can raise the internal body temperature and cause internal muscles—including the bladder—to relax more than they should. Extended exposure to heat can make internal muscles slack and flabby. This German medical text simply states that the old rule of "moderation in all things" applies to temperatures, too, and warns men that *bare feet* and *cold drafts* can lead to illness later on.

I have already covered the importance of fiber in a healthy diet. High-fiber foods are often low in calories and benefit the bowel by aiding digestion and keeping food byproducts from collecting in the bumpy-textured surface of the lower intestine. Other substances are required to "keep the pipes clear," not the least of these being plenty of water throughout the day—at least eight 8-ounce glasses.

But what NOT to do for constipation is just as important as what you do to relieve it. The first impulse when this condition strikes is to reach for a laxative—more than $100 million is spent each year on laxatives and cathartics. There are about 5,000 types of bowel evacuents on the market—some of them being harsh or even poisonous substances that can cause as many problems as they cure.

Mineral oil is the bugaboo of the laxative world—the American Medical Association has been preaching against its use for over 35 years. Although it is an obvious lubricant, it decreases the body's ability to absorb calcium and phosphorus from food. The *mineral oil* itself absorbs vitamins A, D, E, and K, as well as carotene, from the nutrients in the intestines and takes fat-soluble vitamins and minerals from tissues throughout the body. All these valuable substances are then excreted and lost.

Stimulant laxatives like *castor oil* and the chemical *phenolphthalein* work directly on the small intestine to purge out any food matter. These are frequently prescribed by doctors for use prior to medical tests, and their occasional use is not harmful. But frequent purges can cause excess loss of water and body salts, resulting in body weakness. Many popular over-the-counter laxatives are of this type: too harsh for frequent use.

Saline laxatives like *Milk of Magnesia* and *Epsom salts* produce rapid and complete results. The resulting bowel action is so complete, however, that the body may require several days to restart its digestive processing, resulting in "rebound constipation."

Those who feel they must have at least one bowel movement each day may set themselves up for laxative abuse—creating an artificial dependence on laxatives to create a daily evacuation. Overuse of laxatives can lead to *dehydration, malnutrition symptoms, spastic colitis, stomach* and *bowel disorders,* and even *chronic diarrhea.*

There are times when it is wise NOT to take a laxative. Avoid any use if *stomach cramps, nausea, vomiting,* or *fever* is present. These could be symptoms of *appendicitis.* Stimulating your bowels with a laxative could result in rupture of the inflamed organ.

The best treatment for constipation is prevention. Some authorities believe that the most important health maintenance is done on the digestive tract—the body's supply line. Waste material not regularly evacuated from the body can accumulate, and the toxic byproducts of putrefication can be carried by the blood and lymph to every part of the body. There is a strong link between the cleanliness and health of the intestinal tract and the good health of the body as a whole.

Establishing normal intestinal "flora" (natural bacteria that aid in food breakdown) is of primary importance to establishing normal bowel movements. The following kitchen recipe for a *natural food-based laxative* provides a cleansing, revitalizing start to defeating constipation.

NATURAL FOOD ANTIDOTE FOR CONSTIPATION

(ENOUGH FOR ONE PERSON FOR ONE TO TWO WEEKS)

1 cup whey powder

1 1/2 cups brewer's yeast

1 cup wheat germ

1/2 cup psyllium seeds

1/2 cup whole flaxseed

1/2 cup whole mustard seed (optional)

Mix all ingredients together in a large bowl till uniformly blended. Store in a plastic bag or Mason jar.

To use: Place 1 or 2 tablespoons of the mixture in a cup with the beverage of your choice—coffee, tea, milk, juice, or water—and swallow slowly. Always rinse it down with a second glass of your favorite drink. Some users prefer to simply put a spoonful in their mouths and wash it down with plenty of liquid. Take before meals, one to three times daily. Allow a day or two for results—this is not a chemical blast but a gentle food-based laxative.

My father, who was a doctor, used this natural remedy in his practice to treat thousands of constipation cases. It is gentle and shows no negative side effects, and it is without fail a healthy way to evacuate the bowel and create a healthy "internal environment" for ongoing intestinal health.

All the ingredients for this constipation antidote are readily available at health-food stores or co-ops.

New Findings for Prostate Cancer: PC Spes Providing Hope

The dietary supplement PC Spes is a combination of eight Chinese herbs; saw palmetto, licorice, reishi, balkal skullcap, rabdosia, dyers wood, chrysanthemum, and san-qi ginseng. Each of these herbs has been shown in laboratory studies to either kill cancer cells or boost the body's immune system in order to fight cancer. Biochemist Dr. Sophie Chen named her formula "PC" for prostate cancer and "Spes" for the Latin word meaning *hope*. It has turned out that PC Spes *is* giving hope to many men suffering from advanced prostate cancer.

This Chinese herbal blend has been clinically shown to dramatically drop PSA levels, often to undetectable levels. Researchers at the University of California in San Francisco treated 70 patients with PC Spes. Half of the men had never received any type of hormonal therapy, and the other half had developed hormone-resistant prostate cancer. A full 100 percent of the men saw a decline in their PSA levels, and over half of them, 56 percent, had them drop so low that they could no longer be measured. The UCSF team was surprised by how the PSA levels of the group of hormone-resistant men had been affected, with approximately 60 percent of them experiencing more than a 50 percent drop in their levels. In a group of people who had already run through their options, and who were facing the prospect of harsh end-stage chemotherapy, these results are shockingly positive. It appears that PC Spes has promise both as an adjunct therapy in combination with other treatments and as an alternative when others have failed.

Dr. Eric Small of the University of California headed up a study of 33 prostate-cancer patients who were given PC Spes. Again, 100 percent of them saw a major drop in their PSA levels—with 80 percent moving into the undetectable range. One of the men had a bladder mass completely disappear during treatment, and two men with metastasis to the bone saw improvements in their condition.

Although short-term complications, or side effects, of this therapy are considered relatively mild, they should not be overlooked. As is the case with mainstream hormone therapies, PS Spes can cause some breast tenderness and mild breast enlargement. Researchers feel this may be due to the hormonal effects of the formula, which causes the male hormone testosterone to decline in some users. Some men who have not received any prior hormone therapy may experience a decreased libido or a decrease in erections.

It will be several years before any long-term studies can be completed on PC Spes and it must still be considered an experimental therapy. You should, of course, only take the formula under the guidance of a physician. At this time, there is no clear dosage recommendation. The recommended dosages for the UCSF study started with one capsule three times a day, progressed to two capsules three times a day in the second week, and as long as the patients tolerated the treatment moved to three capsules three times a day in the third week and beyond. Others recommend six to 12 capsules a day, depending on the stage of the disease.

The Essiac Story

A product known to help cure hundreds of cancer cases in Canada is now available to the general public.

Its modern use dates to the early decades of the 20th century, when a nurse named Rene Caisse drew thousands of hopeless cancer patients and plenty of medical controversy to her Ontario cancer clinic. Her claim to fame was an herbal therapy she called "Essiac," a series of concoctions she made from a tonic recipe provided by an *Ojibwa Indian* medicine man.

Despite hundreds of documented cures, the Canadian medical

establishment forbade Caisse to practice until she gave up her formula for intensive testing.

Caisse closed her clinic in 1942 but continued to quietly treat those who contacted her for help. A loophole in Canadian law allowed her to dispense the tonic when a patient's doctor gave consent. Rather than sell her healing knowledge to a medical establishment that might forbid its use, she chose to live a modest life, frequently providing her services free of charge to supposedly dying cancer patients, many of whom survived to sing her praises.

Before her death in 1978, Caisse passed on her secrets to a friend, Boston physician Charles Brusch. Before his retirement Brusch was a leading Boston clinician and medical researcher and the personal doctor of President John F. Kennedy. Brusch himself had cancer of the lower bowel, which he said completely disappeared after he used Caisse's formula.

Caisse chose a powerful partner in Brusch. This distinguished doctor didn't hesitate to introduce unheard-of methods to his medical practice, setting trends in polio vaccination, free care for indigent patients, and acupuncture, to name a few areas.

Brusch began administering *Essiac* to his patients in 1959. According to medical records, prostate-cancer patient Wilbur Dymond took the formula for two months. During that time, all hardness in his prostate vanished. He no longer suffered excruciating pain during urination, Brusch reported.

Magazine and newspaper journalists investigated several false "Essiac" formulas that came and went over the years. None were Caisse's own; all of them faded from the market. Finally, with Dr. Brusch's weighty influence, a series of clinical tests were performed using Caisse's recipes. Brusch and his associates learned to heighten and concentrate the medicine's effects and collected hundreds of notarized testimonials to *Essiac's* curative powers.

Unfortunately, the American medical establishment refused to continue cooperating with Brusch's clinical trials unless Caisse gave other researchers her formula for further experiments. When she refused, they labeled *Essiac* "an unknown remedy" and consigned it to its former folk-remedy status.

The late Dr. Brusch joined forces in 1988 with health-radio producer and broadcaster Elaine Alexander, who had impressed him with her extensive research on Essiac. Alexander has made Brusch's updated formula available in stores under the name of *Flor-Essence* (the Canadian Food and Drug Administration forbid use of the name "*Essiac*" because of copyright problems.) You can also find Essiac through a number of on-line resources such as www.harvesthealth.com and www.netrition.com. No prescription is needed to buy the formulas.

When the substance is absorbed into the system, the end result is a slow removal of systemic waste and toxins from the body through a gentle regulation of bowel and urinary-tract functions. Prostate patients who experience painful urine retention frequently find their urine flow gradually increasing to normal. Those with abnormally frequent bathroom visits find themselves returning to a more normal schedule.

Flor-Essence doesn't just treat the prostate. Its makers say it helps almost any problem that involves *inflammation or enlargement of urinary organs*—in men and women. Its tonic effect boosts the immune system, a great help to those undergoing chemical and radiation therapies for cancer, as testified to by Ed Florkoue of Calgary, Alberta. His notarized letter of testimony says the formula relieved his nocturia and dysuria during a long series of radiation treatments for his prostate cancer.

And for the elderly father of Cypriot-Canadian Elli Fletheriou, it proved a cancer cure. Mrs. Fletheriou wrote in a 1993 testimonial letter that her father was diagnosed in October 1992 with a growing prostate cancer. He began taking Flor-Essence immediately and took two bottles along when he went to Cyprus a month later to visit relatives. Three months later, he reported to a Cypriot oncologist for a "tumor checkup." But digital, PSA, and needle biopsy tests found no evidence of cancer.

"We were overwhelmed with surprise at the fast results," Fletheriou wrote. "I still can't believe it worked so fast on my father, who, by the way, is not a very good keeper of health or diet regimens."

Harold Good, a 75-year-old man from Vancouver, Canada, told an investigative reporter from the *Vancouver Sun* about the effectiveness of this cure as a treatment for his prostate problems.

Harold had grown used to rising hourly throughout the night to urinate, "a painful and exhausting ritual" as he termed it. After his wife Peggy experienced a seemingly miraculous cure from ovarian cancer by using an Essiac formula, he decided to try it.

He went to bed early one evening and rose a few hours later "sleep-walking" to relieve himself. Peggy visited the bathroom a few minutes later and was astonished at the gruesome discharge her husband had left behind in the toilet bowl.

"It was a bowl full of pus," she told the reporter. She went to wake Harold, to tell him something was wrong, but he was fast asleep. That was his last late-night bathroom excursion. His prostate hasn't troubled him since, he said. Elaine Alexander, current holder of the secret formula, says its primary ingredients are *slippery-elm bark, burdock root, sheep sorrel,* and *turkey rhubarb root.* Only Alexander and Brusch now know the correct harvesting, handling, and decocting method.

Dr. Jim Chan, a Vancouver naturopath who teaches at a Seattle medical college, says burdock root contains *inulin,* a powerful immune-system modulator. He has used Alexander's tonics to treat cancer patients but cautions against anyone's believing they are the cure-all for cancer. He says that they work best for patients who've had minimal radiation or chemotherapy treatments and that their effectiveness varies from patient to patient.

Caisse herself never claimed to have a sure cancer cure, but her legacy of living patients, Alexander says, speaks for itself.

Like many other powerful medicines, *Flor-Essence* has a healing history traceable to indigenous people. Caisse said she obtained a crude recipe for Essiac from a patient who, in her youth, had treated cases of breast cancer with it. The patient got the remedy in the forests of northern Ontario, from an Ojibwa medicine man. All the herbs contained in the formula are native to Ontario.

There is hope for the hopeless, it would seem, if the testimony of Dr. Brusch is to be believed. As he wrote in his clinical findings, "The results we obtained with thousands of patients of various races, sexes, and ages, with all types of cancer, definitely prove *Essiac* to be a cure for cancer. Studies done in the United States and Canada also fortify this claim."

CHAPTER 10

Impotence:
A Man's Secret Nightmare

"About one out of every 10 men in the United States, from teens to senior citizens, suffers from chronic or continuous impotence," according to the Greater Pittsburgh Impotence Center.

Impotency: The word conjures up nothing but negative associations—and fear that one's sex life is gone forever. Medical authorities define impotency as "the continued failure of a man to achieve and sustain an erection adequate for penetration of the female vagina."

Sex researchers Masters and Johnson describe a man as impotent when his "failure rate approaches 25 percent of his total sexual attempts."

Just look at the words used, all items that strike at the very base of the male ego: *"Failure* to *achieve* or *sustain."*

Inadequate. Unable to achieve. Continued failure. What man would admit to such a condition?

Unfortunately, the vast majority of those men whose prostates are surgically removed or irradiated by radiation are rendered impotent. "Nerve-sparing" prostatectomies preserve potency and are becoming more widespread. But it seems that anytime a man's reproductive organs are affected by illness, impotency can be at least a temporary problem.

Sometimes, impotence occurs when a man simply believes his treatment will make him impotent. In these cases, even when doctors find his "equipment" perfectly intact and functional, the man cannot get an erection.

Before a man concludes he is impotent, he should understand the many outside causes that can interfere with erections. Impotency can be traced back to use of certain medications and prescription drugs, high stress levels, alcohol, disease, and family problems.

Another cause is some mens' unrealistic view of their sex drives. As a man ages, his body reacts differently to sexual stimulation. He may take longer to become aroused and achieve an erection. A 55-year-old whose standard of virility is the average teen-age male is bound to be disappointed in his own perform-ance. Many men don't realize their slowed reactions are natural body changes. They mistakenly believe they are growing impotent. But before I go into the changes you can expect, it's important you know just how an erection works.

More Anatomy

The penis is made of three parallel cylinders, enclosed in an outer sheath of stretchy, elastic skin.

The two major cylinders, called the *corpus cavernosum*, are responsible for the bulk of an erection and provide the familiar rigid, firm shape the penis takes when an erection occurs. These two cylinders of spongy tissue may be compared to long balloons.

When pumped full of blood, they are erect; when not, they are small and limp.

THE PENIS

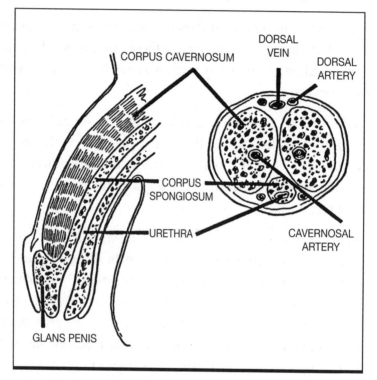

From "BioPotency: A Guide to Sexual Success," by Richard E. Berger, M.D., and Deborah Berger, M.S.W., Rodale Press.

The inside of these cylinders is lined with millions of tiny spongelike caverns called "sinuses." They fill with blood during arousal when the penis is flaccid, however, only enough blood for cell maintenance is present. Millions of tiny sphincters close and open according to incoming stimuli—a complex, intricate system that functions entirely without conscious thought on the male's part. Erection is an involuntary response. Even though some women may not believe it, a man cannot "will an erection."

The third cylinder, called the *corpus spongiosum*, surrounds the urethra—the channel through which semen and urine travel to the outside world. This cylinder also fills with blood during an erection, but it doesn't take on the firmness of its two neighbors. It has another important function to perform.

The *corpus spongiosum* is connected to the *glans penis*, the tip or head of the penis—the organ's most sensitive spot. Those all-important nerves that provide sexual sensation are located here and travel through the *corpus spongiosum* to the spinal cord, which gives erection its "reflexive" character. (So is proven an old adage: It doesn't take any brains to get an erection!)

Mental stimulation results as sensations travel to the brain. All these signals pass back and forth through the *pudendal nerve,* one of a bundle of nerve fibers lying along the *corpus spongiosum.*

Two other sets of nerves, the *sympathetic* and *parasympathetic nerves*, control ejaculation and erection respectively. When sexual arousal becomes intense enough that climax is inevitable, a message travels from the brain down the spinal cord to the sympathetic nerves. This message tells the muscles around the base of the penis to contract rhythmically and release the semen.

Male orgasm is composed of two phases: emission and ejaculation. During sexual arousal, sperm is pumped from the *scrotum* (which encases the testes) through the vas and into the region around the *ejaculatory ducts.* The longer the period of foreplay before climax, the more semen is pumped into the ducts. Emission is the moment called "ejaculatory inevitability." This is when the *seminal vesicles* behind the prostate gland contract and release the seminal fluid.

Ejaculation happens soon afterward, when the muscles surrounding the base of the penis contract powerfully at about one second intervals. The semen is pushed out of the penis with great force. Thus, emission is the collection of seminal fluid and sperm while ejaculation is its elimination. Once emission occurs, it is impossible to voluntarily delay ejaculation.

What Can Go Wrong? Tiny Veins and Squeezing Sinuses

The rigidity, or stiffness, of the penis during an erection comes from an extra spurt of blood into the *corpus cavernosum*. Important arteries supply blood to the "sinuses," which expand and stiffen the organ.

THE PENILE SINUSES: BEFORE ERECTION

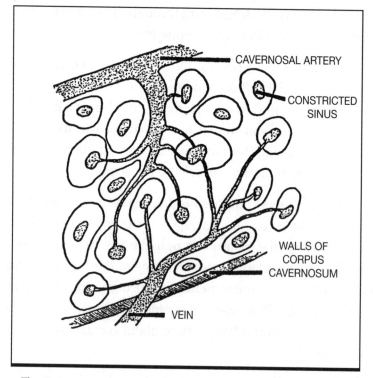

The sinuses are constricted and contain only a small amount of blood when the penis is flaccid.

THE PENILE SINUSES: DURING ERECTION

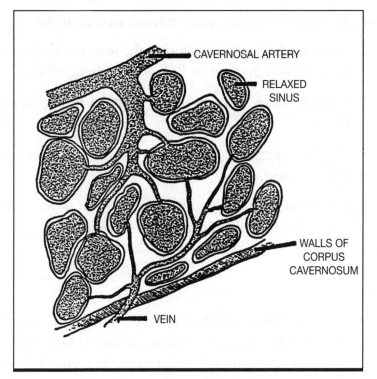

The blood flow increases and the sinuses expand, compressing the veins, when the penis is becoming erect.

From "BioPotency: A Guide to Sexual Success, by Richard E. Berger. M.D. and Deborah Berger, M.S.W., Rodale Press

Tiny thin-walled veins drain blood away from the *sinuses* after climax. These veins are more important than doctors once thought: Dr. Tom Lue, a University of California urologist, has demonstrated that the expanding *sinuses* compress these veins and slow the blood flow out of the penis. But if the veins aren't squeezed tightly enough during erection by the expanding *sinuses*, blood flowing to the penis will simply flow back out through these vein—resulting in either a poorly sustained erection or none at all, much like trying to fill a bathtub without first closing the drain.

There are reasons why these veins may not work properly:

1. Not enough blood is getting to the sinuses. They are not swelling enough to cut off the veins' draining effect.

2. The sinuses are too stiff to be expanded by the incoming blood.

3. The veins are abnormally formed at birth, so they cannot be squeezed shut.

None of these, however, is reason enough to resign yourself to a life of celibacy. Any of them can be successfully treated by a specialist.

Fear

Because erection is such a complicated process, many factors can be involved in its failure. Probably the largest factor is fear. A man's "performance anxiety" can actually influence his sexual ability. John P., a man happily married for 12 years and the father of three children, is a good example.

John's wife Ellen experienced a number of health problems that prompted her doctor to advise against any more pregnancies. He suggested Ellen undergo a *tubal ligation* or John a *vasectomy*.

John, a generous man, felt his wife had undergone enough medical probing. he volunteered to undergo a *vasectomy* in order to "give Ellen a break from the hospital."

John knew vasectomies don't cause impotency—it simply sterilizes a man through removing the *vas deferens*, the path through which sperm travel from the *scrotum*.

But John's father, who had also undergone the surgery, warned his son he was "never the same after that operation."

He never fully explained what he meant. John, though, concluded he must have meant impotency.

John went through with the surgery, despite his misgivings. And after he recovered, he could not get an erection. He had convinced himself, with the help of his father, that he "would not be the same" after the operation.

After two months of therapy, John and Ellen resumed a normal sex life. But not without finding out what a powerful enemy fear can be to a healthy lifestyle.

Even after an erectile problem is "solved," fear of later failure may haunt a man and thus set him up for further disappointments by creating a "self-fulfilling prophecy" of failure.

It's All in Your Head

The brain is man's most potent sex organ. Men can get easily aroused through visual stimulation, but his fear of not being able to perform can lead to erectile problems.

Researchers believe a chemical found in the brain is vital to a man's sex drive. It is called *acetylcholine,* and it supposedly triggers the sex organs' initial reactions to stimuli. If there is a lack of this chemical in the brain, a man rarely thinks of sex and, in fact, will not be stimulated through visual means.

The body makes *acetyicholine* with certain dietary elements— primarily those found in seafood. Those who eat few fish and shellfish might consider a supplement like lecithin, which contains acetylcholine. Lecithin is available in several forms in health-food stores. Authorities recommend about 7,200 milligrams a day for healthy males.

Lecithin is also good for the circulatory system. It breaks cholesterol down into particles small enough to leave the body. If cholesterol cannot escape, it remains in the blood and coats the insides of arteries—literally clogging the blood flow.

Because a man's erection depends on the free flow of blood to his penis, *lecithin* might be a suitable dietary supplement.

Age Changes Things

A man's response to sexual stimulation changes over the years. What some men consider a loss of potency is really only a series of natural changes dictated by age. The changes in no way affect a man's ability to father children or the pleasure he derives from sex.

A recent study of 1,300 American males between 40 and 70 found that 52 percent of them had experienced some sort of impaired sexual performance during the six-month survey period. In fact, approximately 5 perent to 10 percent of males under 40 experience erectile difficulty and 25 percent of men over 50 are impotent.

The younger a man is, the easier and quicker he can achieve an erection. Some men in their late teens and early 20s report they have almost continuous erections, sometimes cause for embarrassment. Jim, for example, recalls his college years.

"I'd be sitting in class with an erection—I'd sometimes have an erection all day long. And it could be embarrassing! You'd have to lose it before you could stand up." A man at his sexual peak—late teens through early 20s—can have intercourse two or three times during a single encounter.

As a man matures into his 30s, his erections will be a little slower. This change, in fact, may produce in him a greater interest in foreplay, which is usually a welcome change as far as his partner is concerned. This man will usually take a little longer to reach orgasm. He may find it easier to control his ejaculation and prolong the pleasure of intercourse for him and his partner.

The climaxes may be slightly less intense, and the quantity of ejaculate may be less, but most men at this age report a deepening enjoyment of sex as a form of lovemaking and intimacy.

As a man reaches his 50s or 60s, even more time is needed to attain a firm erection. This doesn't mean the man is losing his ability to make love. No one should panic when these changes become apparent. Foreplay simply becomes more essential. Often, the penis will need to be caressed to achieve a full erection.

Older men do not respond to visual stimulation the way they did at age 18. George was 65 when he took his potency concerns to his doctor.

"Nothing happens down there," he told the doctor. "I used to be able to get hard just by looking at a pretty girl. My wife is still quite pretty, and in the past I've always been able to just look at her and get an erection. I'm still really attracted to her, but I look at her and nothing happens. I can watch her getting undressed; I feel excited, but my penis just lies there."

George's problem was solved with a little help from his still pretty wife, who was glad to help him with a little direct stimulation and the addition of magnesium, zinc, and B vitamins in his diet. Their doctor helped George to "get real" with his expectations: Erections for men his age don't have the texture, urgency, or forceful ejaculation of youngsters'. But what they lose in texture they gain in staying power.

Probably the most noticeable and disturbing feature of the aging process is the increase in "latency periods"—the periods of time between successive ejaculations. For some men in their 60s, it may be hours before they can attain another erection. While this may prevent intercourse during the interval, it may provide more time for other forms of sexual activity.

None of these changes should be interpreted as a sign of impotency. They are simply changes in the ways the male body responds to sexual stimulation. Taken in stride, they offer opportunities to broaden the kinds of pleasure one can receive from sexual relations.

OTHER CAUSES OF IMPOTENCY:

Medication

It's hard to find a man over age 40 who isn't on some kind of regular prescription medication. Prescription drugs can be potency killers—especially those used to control high blood pressure. Some men's sexual performance declines dramatically after they begin taking blood-pressure medication, but many simply attribute the loss to "old age," never considering the effect the medicine may have.

Other drugs that commonly affect potency include barbiturates, tranquilizers, reserpine, narcotics, antihistamines, antidepressants, and amphetamines—alone or in combination with other chemicals. Controlled substances like marijuana and cocaine—including "crack"—may also steal away potency. The obvious solution is to consult with your doctor. If your health permits, suspect drugs should be temporarily stopped or alternatives found.

DRUGS THAT MAY AFFECT POTENCY

GENERIC NAME	BRAND NAME	GENERIC NAME	BRAND NAME
Blood pressure medicines/diuretics		**Major tranquilizers**	
Thiazides	Diuril, Esidrix, Hygroton and others	Fluphenazine	Prolixin
		Trifluoperazine	Stelazine
		Prochlorperazine	Compazine
Spironolactone	Aldactone	Mesoridazine	Serentil
*Hydralazine	*Apresoline	Promazine	Sparine
*Minoxidil	*Loniten	Chlorpromazine	Thorazine
Methyldopa	Aldomet	Thioridazine	Mellaril
Clonidine	Catapres	Haloperidol	Haldol
Reserpine	Serpasil, Sandril	Droperidol	Innovar
Guanethidine	Ismelin	Thiothixene	Navane
Bethanidine		Chloprothixine	Taractan
Phenoxybenzamine	Dibenzaline		
Antidepressants		**Drugs for irregular heartbeats**	
		Disopyramide	Norpace
Nortriptyline	Aventyl	Phentolamine	Regitine
Amitriptyline	Elavil	*Prazosin	*Minipress
Desipramine	Norpramine	Propanolol	Inderal
Doxepin	Sinequan	Metaprolol	Lopressor
Imipramine	Tofranil	* Least likely to cause potency problems	
Isocarboxazide	Marplan		
Phenelzine	Nardil	**Drugs for bladder or bowel spasms**	
Tranylcypromine	Parnate	Propantheline bromide	Pro-Banthine
Pargylene	Eutonyl	Atropine (usually used in combination with other drugs)	
Furazolidone	Furoxone		
Procarbazine	Matulane		
Lithium Carbonate		**Drugs for Parkinson's Disease**	
Anxiety medications		Biperidin	Akineton
		Cycrimine	Pagitane
Chlordiazepoxide	Librium	Procyclidine	Kenadrin
Oxazepam	Serax	Trihexyphenidyl	Artane
Diazepam	Valium	Benztropine	Cogentin
Chlorazepate	Tranxene	Levodopa	Larodopa, Sinemet
Meprobamate	Miltown Equanil		
Tybamate	Tybatran		

continued

DRUGS THAT MAY AFFECT POTENCY
Continued

GENERIC NAME	BRAND NAME

Drugs for allergies and motion sickness (antihistimines)

Dimenhydrinate	Dramamine
Diphenhydramine	Benadryl
Hydroxyzine	Vistaril
Meclizine	Antivert, Bonine
Promethazine	Phenergan

Muscle relaxants

Cyclobenzaprine	Flexeril
Orphenadrine	Norflex

COMMONLY ABUSED DRUGS

Alcohol
Amphetamines
Barbituates
Cocaine
Marijuana
Narcotics (such as heroin and morphine)
Nicotine
Opiates

GENERIC NAME	BRAND NAME

Miscellaneous drugs

Cimetidine	Tagamet (for ulcers)
Clofibtate	Altromid-S (for high cholesterol and high fat in the blood)
Cyproterone acetate	(a horomone used to treat certain types of cancer)
Digoxin	Lanoxin (for heart problems)
Epsilon aminocaproic acid	Amicar (for abnormal bleeding)
Estrogens	(female horomones used to treat prostate cancer)
Glucocorticoids	(horomones used to treat severe allergies, asthma and other breathing problems, arthritis, lupus and other diseases)
Immunosuppressive agents	(agents sometimes used to treat arthritis and lupus; used by transplant patients to prevent tissue rejection)
Indomethacin	Indocin (mainly for arthritis)
Methysergide	Sansert (for headache relief)
Metoclopramide	Reglan (for heartburn)
Metronidazole	Flagyl (for infections)
Phenytoin	Dilantin (for seizures)
Progestins	(female horomones used to treat certain types of cancer)

Source: Drugs and Male Sexual Dysfunction. American Urological Association Update Series. (Houston: American Urological Association, 1984).

If you take medication and are experiencing erectile difficulty, keep these considerations in mind:

- A variety of drugs can cause erection problems. Some anti-depressants, including *Prozac*, *Zoloft*, and *Paxil*, have been found to be problematic.

- Different men have differing degrees of sensitivity to drugs. One man may lose his potency because of a certain medication, while another man taking an identical dosage will maintain full functioning.

- Drugs interact with each other. A man may take a single drug and experience no problems, but when he adds another medication, he may develop erectile problems.

- The body's tolerance for medication may change with time. A medication taken for years without effect may suddenly steal away potency.

Alcohol

Overindulging in alcohol can cause erectile difficulty. If the drinking is only occasional, the difficulty usually passes away with the intoxication.

But those who indulge may frequently find their reflexes and sensory ability impaired over the long-term. Their organisms may become less intense and sex may lose its savor.

Alcoholics may find they have erection problems even when they are "on the wagon." A heavy drinker may even permanently impair his ability to make love. Alcohol can damage the testicles' ability to produce testosterone. The liver damage that accompanies alcohol abuse changes the way the body uses testosterone. This adds up to a decreased sexual desire and an inability to achieve or maintain an erection.

Many alcoholics who seek treatment for impotence are given hormone shots to increase their testosterone levels, but this therapy isn't always successful. Those whose metabolism is permanently impaired sometimes report mild breast development and a softening of facial hair: Their bodies convert the testosterone into female hormones

One or two drinks may increase one's libido by loosening inhibitions and lessening stress. But anyone interested in a long, healthy sex life is well advised to imbibe in spirits only moderately.

Smoking and Environmental Factors

Research is beginning to point the finger at tobacco as a cause of male impotency. Evidence links smoking to *hardening of the arteries*, including those vessels vital to erection. When penile and *pubic arteries* harden and narrow, they are unable to expand enough to allow sufficient blood into the *corpus cavernosum* to cause an erection.

In most men, this condition develops over many years. Smoking cigarettes today may not affect your sex life. But research indicates this may be the case for a few highly sensitive men. Among them, smoking may indeed cause erectile problems before the arteries are damaged.

A 1994 study of Vietnam veterans published in the *American Journal of Epidemiology* showed that 3.7 percent of the current smokers suffered from impotency as opposed to 2.2 percent of nonsmokers in the group. In addition, according to a spokesman for the manufacturer of the impotency drug Viagra, 75 percent of the men in the company's clinical trials were in fact current or former smokers.

Secondarily, smoking can contribute to *bladder cancer*, which, unfortunatly, frequently requires surgery. Many bladder surgeries leave the patient impotent.

Doctors find that other environmental pollutants found in the workplace may also affect patients sexually. People who work with toxic chemicals, thinners, lead, and other heavy metals frequently report erectile difficulty.

Diabetes and Chronic Diseases

Impotency is a classic first symptom of diabetes, a common metabolic disorder that can wait until later in life to strike. Loss of sexual function may be due to a combination of blood-vessel changes and disorders of the nerves that connect the penis to the spinal cord.

Dr. Isadore Rossman details its symptoms in *Looking Forward*, a text on aging. He says that failure to have erections during the night, on awakening, or during masturbation indicates an organic basis for the impotency—it's not just psychological.

Rossman estimates that up to 50 percent of male diabetics develop impotency. Damaged nerves prevent sexual impulses from being transmitted to the valves of the penis. Even with abundant sexual stimulation, the message cannot get through, the valves remain closed, and blood is unable to enter the penis and produce an erection.

Similar problems may be experienced by men with vascular and neural impairments not related to diabetes. These problems are sometimes difficult for doctors to detect, but they are more obvious in men whose nerve pathways were affected by previous surgery or by head or spinal injuries. Degenerative nerve disorders like multiple sclerosis and spina bifida may also effect potency.

Those with *chronic fatigue syndrome, mononucleosis, heart disease* or *stroke, genital* or *venereal disease, high blood pressure, emphysema,* or *severe lower-back pain,* may also suffer from impotency.

Those with *neural* and *vascular disorders* are ready patients for modern and old-fashioned impotency cures detailed later in this chapter. But prevention is the best cure: Those at risk for diabetes—black men, for example, and anyone with a family history of the disease—should carefully control their intake of sugary and high-fat foods.

Depression

Chronic depression is common among men in their middle and older years—when unmet youthful expectations haunt the less than successful and personal-fulfillment issues plague those who've made it to the top. *Depression* wears away at sexual desire. Its effect on *serotonin,* a brain chemical that regulates coping skills is well documented. Depression may also throw off secretions of *testosterone* and *thyroid secretions.*

Counseling and a round of antidepressant medication may be required for relief. *Testosterone* may act as a supplement and/or powerful placebo for some men whose self-doubts are augmented by sexual problems.

Endocrine Disorders

Your glands can take away your potency. The *thyroid, pituitary,* and *adrenal glands* can all play roles in impotency. Talk about these with your doctor, and check your family's health history for relatives who may have suffered from too much or not enough of any of these secretions. Simple hormone imbalances may also affect potency.

Stress

Loss of a loved one or a job, finding a parking spot, or getting a big promotion—all create their own forms of anxiety that can put the kibosh on sexual functions. Whether negative or positive, your body responds to losses, responsibilities, or almost any change with a rush of blood to the limbs—a good way to escape. The cumulative effect of these daily stresses can be impotence. Your blood is in your arms and legs, set to help you fight an enemy or run away. It's not in your central body, where it can easily flow "southward."

It may be impossible to eliminate some stresses, but if you learn to relax, slow down and say "no" to extra projects, you may find your sex life improving.

Determining the Cause

In recent years, great strides have been made in the diagnosis of impotency. Sometimes the cause is obvious—*prostatectomy*, an *injury*, *birth defects*, and *drug reactions* are easily detected.

Those with more "mysterious" ailments may undergo some of the diagnostic tests commonly used by doctors. This is only a brief outline, however; your doctor will have more detailed descriptions of his diagnostic tools.

Blood and *urine tests* detect abnormal hormone, protein, or body-chemical levels that can indicate specific problems.

Cystoscopy is the use of a special viewing scope to assess the bladder and prostate.

Corporacavernosogram is an X-ray method that frequently reveals conditions of restricted blood flow to the *corporum cavernosum*—the balloonlike erectile tissues.

Penile arteriograms create a "map" of the blood vessels in and around the penis. Doctors can sometimes see blockages or damaged tissues and pinpoint where the problem lies.

Cystometrogram (CMG) or *electromyogram* (EMG) tests are sometimes performed on the bladder. They test nerve and muscle functions that may influence the penis.

The bulbocavernosus reflex latency time (BC Reflex) *test* and *biothesiometry* indicate whether the penile nerve supply is normal for erection.

The nocturnal penile tumescence test (NPT) determines whether the cause of impotency is physical or psychological. The doctor uses a gauge or monitor to check the automatic erections every man has periodically as he sleeps. If these do not occur, the impotency probably has a physical cause.

WHAT CAN BE DONE?

Sex Therapy

Many impotency patients whose conditions were called physical regained their sexual vigor through a standard course of sex therapy—sitting down and talking with a trained counselor, using visualization and relaxation exercises, and enlisting the help of a supportive partner. In a study cited by Dr. Anne Simons in her book *Before You Call the Doctor*, a large group of men with "diabetic erection loss" were treated with a standard sex-therapy course. Almost all regained their erections. Some statistics give sex therapists an 80 percent success rating in treating erectile problems.

Seeing a therapist doesn't mean you are mentally ill or somehow inferior. You go to a doctor to get better when you are ill, don't you? Many of the therapy "exercises" are truly fun—one learns how to concentrate less on the penile sensations and generalize pleasure throughout the body through touching and sensual massage, just to name one option.

Yohimbine Therapy

If standard sex therapy doesn't work, the doctor may prescribe yohimbine—a drug that is derived from the bark of an African tree and has legendary aphrodisiac properties. About one-third of the men who try this drug report increased erections, but its effectiveness seems to fade after a year or more of use. It works by stimulating blood flow to the penis.

Papaverine and Prostaglandin Injections

Many diabetics who are accustomed to injecting themselves with insulin make good use of *papaverine*—a "high-octane" drug that is injected into the penis before sex. The drug relaxes penile blood vessels allowing more blood to flow into the *corpus cavernosum*. *Papaverine* works within 10 minutes, and the resulting erection can last an hour or more. *Prostaglandin* is another vein dilator in common use. Some men use these medications for years, but others shy away from their use because they'te frightened at the prospect of wielding a needle in such a delicate area.

Vacuum Constriction

One popular option is a vacuum-constriction device, a plastic cylinder attached to a pump. The cylinder is placed over the flaccid penis before lovemaking, and the vacuum draws blood into the penis. A band is then put at the base of the erection, trapping the blood inside.

Almost 90 percent of the men who use these devices are

satisfied with them. Manufacturers usually supply instructional videotapes and toll-free numbers to guide beginners.

But vacuum devices don't suit some others. Spontaneous sex is impossible, and the device is somewhat cumbersome to use.

THE INFLATABLE PENILE PROSTHESIS

RESERVOIR FILLED WITH SALINE SOLUTION

PUMP

CYLINDERS IMPLANTED IN ERECTILE TISSUE ON THE UNDERSIDE OF THE PENIS

Penile Implants

A surgical option chosen each year by about 20,000 men—a small minority—is the penile implant, a surgically installed prosthesis that makes the penis rigid enough for intercourse.

Some simpler implants are made of flexible, semi-rigid material—creating in effect, a permanent erection. Others are inflatable implants that are flaccid when not in use but can be "stimulated" into erection through a squeeze bulb hidden in the scrotum.

Another "inflatable" device uses hydraulic cylinders implanted in the penis. A fluid reservoir is placed in the abdomen and provides a saline "filling" for the erection when the man pumps a squeeze bulb.

Hinged and "malleable" prostheses are also used by some doctors, but they are waning in popularity.

Prosthetic implantation is a relatively simple surgery, requiring an hour or less under general anesthesia. Recovery takes two weeks or so, and sex can resume in four to eight weeks after surgery.

A Simpler Life

Some men opt to forgo all the hardware and pharmaceuticals and simply learn to live with their impotence. They say they are just happy to be alive and free of cancer and pain, with or without sex. They find a fulfilling life through work, recreation, and relationships that are free of sexual complications.

CHAPTER 11

Food and Supplements for a Richer Sex Life

Before you read or believe anything in this chapter, be aware that the federal Food and Drug Administration says there is no such thing as an aphrodisiac.

An aphrodisiac is a substance reported by some to improve sexual vitality and performance. Laws expressly forbid manufacturers to make claims of sexual potency for their products, because their claims usually don't live up to the stringent pharmaceutical tests required by the FDA.

But man's centuries-old pursuit of bigger and better erections continues. The legendary attributes of some substances have produced some off-the-wall results: Poachers continue to deplete Africa's herds of white rhinoceroses—in the Orient, the creatures' ground-up horns are believed to improve sexual performance. Other legendary "aphrodisiacs" include ground pearls, mandrake roots worn around the neck, ginger-root tea, baths in special hot springs, and quarts of oysters, downed raw and chased with beer.

Let us take a moment to explore some of the world's more enduring stories of potent flora and fauna, in the hope that some of the less exotic claims about "aphrodisiacs" may have a grain of reality among the clouds of legend.

The *Anango-Ranga*, an Indian holy book, contains several recipes specially designed to increase male sexual vigor.

Some foods that appear repeatedly are *cucumbers, beans, sugar, asparagus, eggs, onions, garlic,* and *honey.*

One recipe claims thqat "the patient, no matter what his age, will retain vigor and be able to enjoy 100 women." The ambitious man should combine 150 grains of fiber from the *Moh tree (bassia latefolia)* with cow's milk, the *Anango-Ranga* says.

Scientists say the pith of the Moh tree contains up to 58 percent fermentable sugar—a ready source of energy. Honey would provide a good substitute effect.

Ginseng is another substance long touted for its sexual powers. Its scientific name *Panax notoginseng* is derived from the Greek *Panax,* meaning "all-healing," and the Chinese *Schinseng,* meaning "man-root." The root of the *ginseng* plant sometimes resembles the human body. It is native to China, Korea, and Siberia, but its most potent varieties grow wild in the United States.

Along with its aphrodisiac qualities, the *ginseng root* is also credited with rebuilding tissues, stimulating energy, and strengthening the body against mental and physical stress.

Ginseng isn't cheap, and it can be difficult to store while retaining its effectiveness. *Ginseng tea* is available in loose or bag forms at supermarkets, however, and stronger *ginseng drinks* can be found in most health markets and catalogs.

The Chinese have long believed that *Bird's-nest Soup* is a powerful aphrodisiac. The soup is traditionally made from the nests of sea swallows. They contain large amounts of mineral-laden edible *seaweed* and phosphorus-rich *fish spawn*.

Caviar, too, has been noted through history as a sexual stimulant. Legend holds that Empress Catherine the Great of Russia could not produce an heir with her husband, despite many attempts. She therefore ate several pounds of *caviar* and soon conceived. (She also employed the services of a captain of the Royal Guard, whose *caviar* consumption went unrecorded.)

But *caviar* is expensive, a luxury by anyone's standards. Few can afford to eat it by the pound. The following recipe makes a tasty spread for morning toast or an evening snack eaten on crackers. It contains only tablespoons of the "black gold," but some say that's plenty enough to stimulate the desired effect.

POTENT CAVIAR SPREAD

2 tablespoons minced pimento

2 tablespoons anchovy paste

2 tablespoons minced chives or green onion

1 teaspoon lemon juice

3 tablespoons caviar

Mix thoroughly; refrigerate covered for at least 30 minutes before serving.

Those who still cannot stomach caviar's price tag may want to try herring roe, a less-expensive substitute, credited with the creation of thousands of Russian and Ukrainian peasant children.

H E R R I N G   R O E   S P R E A D

2 cans soft herring roe

1 ounce butter

2 sliced tomatoes

3 small fried potatoes

1/4 cup flour

4 slices cucumber

a dash of salt

2 slices of toast

Roll the herring roe in the flour and fry lightly in butter. Sprinkle with salt. Serve on toast and top with cucumber and tomato slices with the potatoes as a side dish.

Oysters are also legendary restorers of male potency. American railroad magnate and gourmand "Diamond Jim" Brady was said to have an enormous appetite for *oysters* on the halfshell—and for pretty actresses too. This is a try-it-at-home recipe for those interested in exploring this option:

O Y S T E R   B E D   S A L A D

2 dozen oysters, half-shelled or shucked

1 beet root, cooked and sliced

2 tomatoes, cut into chunks

1 cup raw carrot, grated

1/2 cup onion, sliced thin

1/2 teaspoon lemon juice (optional)

olives

salt and pepper to taste

4 large lettuce leaves

Arrange ingredients attractively on the lettuce leaves and sprinkle with lemon juice. If you prefer, cut up the lettuce and toss it in a bowl with the other ingredients, using the lemon as a dressing.

Naturopathic doctors have discovered a few substances they say have direct and positive effects on sexual functions. A few are listed here:

Gotu-kola: This is a Chinese herb reported to be able to keep old age at bay. Those who drink gotu-kola tea supposedly stay vital well into their 80s and 90s. The herb is a hormonal tonic. It has a soothing effect on the nervous system and also aids in digestion, experts say.

Licorice: I'm referring here not to the gummy black candies sold at old-time movie houses but to a Chinese variation on the strong-flavored herb. Herbalists say the licorice plant contains more than 100 medicinal compounds. A legendary sexual stimulant, licorice is combined with milk and honey to boost male sexual desires. Licorice is also thought to be helpful in treating high cholesterol, inflammations, wounds, fevers, and allergies.

Kavakava: This is made from the root of the Piper methsyticum, a shrub native to the islands of the South Pacific. Natives scrape the roots and cut them into pieces, which are either chewed like gum or added to food. Consumed internally, the natives believe, kavakava steps up the sex drive of men or women. Moreover, when kavakava oil is spread on the tip of the penis, it controls premature ejaculation, natives say.

Sarsaparilla: The root of this plant, native to tropical America, has been said to contain testosterone, the hormone responsible for the human sex drive. Perhaps the movie cowboy who ordered a sarsaparilla soda in the Old West saloon wasn't such a sissy, after all.

A European Cure for the Impotent

Ongoing research in Europe has found that *O.K.A.S. peptide*, a formulation of enzymes that encourage hormone production, is a useful tool in restarting one's sexual fire.

Elena Groth, a European naturopath who specializes in difficult cases of impotency, found a direct correlation between impotency and a man's unconscious erections during sleep. Specialists have long suspected that hormonal imbalances play a vital role in impotency.

But Groth found that users of the *O.K.A.S. peptide* formulation had nocturnal erections that lasted up to 50 percent longer than normal. She surmised that prolonged use of the formula slowly corrects hormone imbalances, which in turn normalizes erections. The effect works itself into the waking world, where a formerly impotent man can put the healing to use during sexual intercourse. Best results are obtained by men over age 50 who have suffered extended bouts of impotency.

Test results show this natural supplement has no noticeable side effects. It works well for men whose doctors can find no physical reason for their impotency. Light exercise seems to heighten the effects.

Joe H. was 49 when he decided to give up on sex—it wasn't worth the frustration and humiliation anymore. For reasons no doctor could detect, he could not achieve an erection.

Joe's wife told him she would love him no matter what, but Joe felt robbed of a vital part of his manhood.

During a visit to his natural-food store for multivitamins, Joe picked up a trial bottle of O.K.A.S. peptide, figuring he had nothing to lose in trying.

Within a month, Joe and his wife were able to make love again. His ego was restored as well, he said.

Hospital tests have shown that *O.K.A.S. peptide* is also effective in treating hormone variations in women, especially those experiencing troublesome menopause.

The formulation has the curious effect of stimulating the ovaries as well. Groth has had a measure of success in treating cases of female infertility via *O.K.A.S. peptide* in combination with other "female" herbs.

Because *peptide formulations* are a bit expensive, many Europeans like to supplement them with muira-puama, an herb that seems to work in synergy with peptides, boosting their effectiveness.

Another unique healing combination from overseas is especially effective in cases in which impotence is linked with prostate problems. It is a combination of *beta sitosterol, campesterol,* and *stigmasterol,* all of which normalize prostate functions.

Sometimes called "BCS," these natural ingredients can aid in prostate and impotency problems via an all-vegetable formula that is approved even for strict vegetarians. It is a proven cholesterol control, that works by suspending bile in the bloodstream and opening the bile duct and other glandular sphincters. It is now widely available on the United States health-food market.

The Danes also contribute their bit toward the war on impotency with a herb and vitamin program called *LV therapy*.

This combination was developed by Flemming Norgaard, a Danish M.D. Patients who took his formula said *rheumatic pains, herpes viruses, angina pain,* and "the tiring effect of old age" were relieved after a month or two of the supplement.

Norgaard said this isn't medicine: He said it's a food supplement that aids in cell growth and function. It contains several compounds I've already discussed, including *antioxidants, pumpkinseed, minerals, vitamin A,* and several healing herbs. Because of its health-giving effects patients say, their immune systems are strengthened. They get fewer colds, have more energy, and maintain better dispositions!

LV's favorable effect on the urinary tract isn't the least of its powers. Taken regularly, it helps bladder and urethra disorders and keeps them from returning. It aids in curing even stubborn cases or incontinence.

Prostate sufferers also swear by *LV's* effectiveness, especially when it is used along with other cures. It normalizes prostate functions and can help relieve stress and depression associated with disease or illness. The sense of well-being some men experience with its use can act as a natural aphrodisiac.

Damiana, an herb recommended for prostate relief, is truly a powerful aphrodisiac, according to Dr. Zofchak of Pennsylvania. He recommends taking the herb with *saw palmetto,* another natural substance that forestalls any irritation to the urinary tract and sexual organs.

Saffron, a bright-yellow, expensive herb from India, also is legendary as an aphrodisiac. Because it can be very dangerous in large doses, the editors of *Prevention* magazine recommend taking *riboflavin* supplements instead. Analysis of the *saffron flower* reveals high levels of this important vitamin, which aids in hydrogen transport among cells. It helps to break down fatty acids and aids in removing toxins from nerve cells.

Many scientists believe that time-honored aphrodisiacs work on the simple *placebo principal*—if you believe it will work, it will. But most agree that the best sexual tonic is good health. Try a good, low-fat diet, plenty of sleep, and light exercise and see if that regimen won't boost your libido!

Glossary

Acute: a condition characterized by a sudden onset of symptoms and a sharp rise in symptoms. Duration is usually short.

Androgens: hormones responsible for development and maintenance of male sex characteristics. Testosterone is an androgen. An absence of androgens will usually cause the prostate gland to shrink.

Atrophy: the wasting or shrinking in size of tissues or organs

Balloon dilation: a benign prostatic hypertrophy treatment also called *transurethral dilation*, it uses a catheter with a special balloon tip. While within the prostate, the balloon is inflated to enlarge the passage for urine flow.

Benign: a term used to describe a nonmalignant growth that does not invade or destroy neighboring tissue.

Benign prostatic hypertrophy (BPH): enlargement or growth of the glandular tissue of the prostate, it typically begins around age 40. This is NOT cancer; it does not invade or attack neighboring cells. The condition may cause the prostate to grow against the urethra and compress the bladder outlet, causing voiding difficulty.

Biological therapy: an experimental cancer therapy based on boosting the body's own resistance to cancer. Substances under study include the colony-stimulating factor (which stimulates white blood-cell production) and interferons and interleukins (body proteins that fight infection).

Biopsy: removal of a small amount of tissue from an organ or gland for study and diagnosis. It's most commonly used to determine if cancer is present.

Bladder: an elastic sac that stores the urine before it is removed from the body through the urethra

Brachytherapy: a radiation therapy that uses implanted radioactive pellets or "seeds." It's also called interstitial radiation.

Carcinogens: cancer-causing agents

Catheter: a hollow, flexible tube that is passed through the urethra into the bladder to drain off urine. It is used during and after surgery or whenever a patient cannot urinate normally.

Chronic: a term that describes a condition that lasts or recurs over a long time. Some diseases are chronic because they progress slowly or symptoms persist for a long time.

Corpus cavernosum: two long cylinders located in the penis, which fill with blood and provide rigidity during an erection

Corpus spongiosum: a cylindrical channel that passes between the corpus cavernosum. It provides a channel for the nerve bundle that gives the penis tip its sensitivity.

Cystoscopy: examination of the urinary tract through a special viewing tube. It's used to help find urinary obstructions.

Dysuria: difficult or painful urination. It be a symptom of prostate disorders.

Ejaculation: discharge or expulsion of semen from the penis, usually accompanied by an orgasm. The ejaculate fluid, or semen, consists of sperm and other secretions.

Ejaculatory ducts: tubes that connect the seminal vesicles to the prostate and the urethra

Epididymis: a long, convoluted tube that winds along the back edge of each testicle. Sperm are stored in the epididymis until they reach maturity.

Erection: enlargement and stiffening of the penis as a result of sexual stimulation.

Essential fatty acids: Nutritional acids that help maintain the elasticity of cell tissues

Estrogen: a general name for female hormones, which are responsible for the development of reproductive organs and secondary sex characteristics in females. It was once used for prostate cancer treatment.

Fertile: capable of conceiving children.

Flow cytometry: a procedure used to measure the

amount of genetic material within a biopsied cell sample. These samples help doctors plan cancer treatments.

High-energy radiation: a therapy that uses radiation accelerators like neutrons, protons, and helium ions to irradiate cancer growths

Hormone therapy: a prostate-cancer treatment that uses female hormones to reduce production of testosterone, which is needed for prostate-cancer reproduction.

Hyperthermia: another word for "heat." Hyperthermia therapy uses microwave heat, applied to the entire body or to a specific area, to shrink cancer cells.

Hypertrophy: excessive development or growth of an organ or gland

Impotence: inability in the male to achieve and maintain an erection sufficient for penetration of a female vagina

Incontinence: inability to control bladder or bowel functions.

Macrobiotics: a method of extending one's life span and avoiding disease through diet and lifestyle in harmony with the environment.

Masturbation: stimulation or manipulation of one's own genitals for sexual gratification

Metastasis: the spread of cancer cells to other, unaffected parts of the body

Nephritis: acute or chronic kidney inflammation. It's sometimes a result of stagnation of urine due to untreated prostate problems.

Nocturia: an urge or need to urinate at night

Nodule: a small mass of tissue or a tumor, generally malignant

Oncogene therapy: potential cancer therapy that replaces defective genes with healthy ones

Orgasm: the climax of the sexual act. It is accompanied by muscular contractions, release of tension, and pleasurable sensations. In men, orgasm is usually accompanied by ejaculation. Orgasm may occur without an erection.

Parasympathetic nerves: the system of nerves responsible for penile erections.

Penile prostheses: implants placed in the penis that allow simulation of a natural erection. They are usually used by men rendered impotent through illness, surgery, hormones, or radiation treatments.

Penis: the male sexual and urinary excretory organ

Potency: the ability to achieve and maintain an erection sufficient for vaginal penetration.

Potency-sparing technique: a variation on the radical open prostatectomy, in which the nerves and blood vessels responsible for erection are left in place. Doctors find this unfeasible when the tumor is large or has spread throughout the prostate.

Prostate gland: a chestnut-sized gland located directly below the male bladder and surrounding a portion of the urethra. It secretes a fluid component of semen, which is expelled during ejaculation.

Prostate specific antigen: a blood protein produced by the growth of prostate cells. A PSA blood test can usually detect prostate cancer through measurements of this protein in the blood.

Prostatitis: acute or chronic inflammation of the prostate, usually caused by an infection, congestion, or irritation

Pudendal nerves: nerves responsible for carrying sexual sensations from the penis to the spinal cord and then to the brain. These nerves are frequently cut during abdominal prostate surgeries.

Resectoscope: a surgical instrument inserted into the penis during transurethral prostatectomy. It "resections," or cuts away, the prostate tissue interfering with urinary function.

Retrograde: a term describing a condition in which sperm goes backward into the bladder instead of being propelled forward and out of the end of the penis. This is frequently a harmless result of some prostate operations.

Scrotum: the external skin sac that contains the testicles

Selenium: a trace element needed to preserve cell elasticity and improve the supply of oxygen to the heart.

Seminal fluid (semen): a thick yellowish-white fluid that contains spermatozoa. It is a mixture of secretions from the testicles, seminal vesicles, prostate, and

Cowper's gland designed to deliver healthy sperm cells to the female reproductive system.

Seminal vesicles: two folded glandular structures that lie against the lower rear of the bladder. They provide sperm with a high-energy milk sugar, a component of the semen.

Sigmoidoscope: a viewing instrument about 10 inches long. It is sometimes introduced into the anus as part of a rectal examination.

Sperm, or Spermatozoa: the male sex cell or gamete that carries the male genetic information and strives to fertilize the female ovum and create new life. It is a component of semen ejaculated from the penis.

Stent: a tiny tubular device made of surgical metal or plastic. Surgeons use this experimental implant to relieve prostate-gland obstruction and shore up the neck of the bladder.

Sterile: unable to produce offspring.

Suprapubic/retropubic Prostatectomy: surgical procedures by which all or part of the prostate is removed through an abdominal incision

Sympathetic nerves: set of nerves in a male responsible for control of ejaculation.

Testicles: two male reproductive glands that are enclosed in the scrotum. The testicles, or testes, produce sperm and androgens.

Testosterone: a male hormone that triggers prostate growth and other forms of sexual maturation at puberty.

It also triggers the male and female sex drives. Doctors have found that its presence promotes the growth and spread of prostate-cancer cells.

Transrectal ultrasound: a diagnostic tool that uses sound waves to create a computer image of the prostate. A doctor inserts an instrument into the rectum that bounces sound waves off the prostate, revealing areas of abnormal growth.

Transurethral prostatectomy: surgical removal of prostate tissue via a resectoscope through the penis rather than an abdominal incision. Transurethral incision of the prostate (TUIP) uses a similar system to remove the core of the prostate. Transurethral ultrasound-guided laser-induced prostatectomy (TULIP) uses ultrasound to guide the resectoscope and a high-energy laser beam to remove interfering tissue.

Tumor: a swelling or enlargement due to abnormal tissue growth. Tumors grow faster than neighboring tissues and serve no useful purpose. They can be benign (harmless) or malignant (cancerous).

Uremia: a toxic excess of urine and other wastes in the blood. These wastes are usually processed through the kidneys. Uremia may be a symptom of prostate trouble.

Urethra: the muscular tube through which urine passes from the bladder and out of the body. In men, both urine and seminal fluid pass through the urethra.

Urine: waste fluid excreted by the kidneys, stored in the bladder, and expelled through the urethra. Urine is 96 percent water and 4 percent dissolved waste substances.

Urology: the study, diagnosis, and treatment of diseases of the genitourinary tract

Vas deferens: one of two tubes attached to the epididymis, extending to the prostate and looping upward behind the bladder. It carries mature sperm through several developmental steps and glands before delivering it to the urethra for ejaculation to the outside.

Zinc: a trace mineral essential for reproductive health. Zinc deficiency has been linked to prostatitis and impotency in men.

· A P P E N D I X   I ·

Groups and Organizations That Can Help

No man need suffer alone when dealing with prostate problems, cancer, or impotence. Many medical organizations, self-help groups, and support services exist for the man or wife willing to take the first step.

Several studies show that men who seek support recover more quickly from surgery. Of those with cancer, a Stanford University study found that support-group members lived an average of 36 months after joining the group. Men who didn't join usually lived about 18 months. Group members had a better outlook on life, doctors said, and were less moody, fatigued, and depressed.

For up-to-date information on cancer, BPH, support groups. and other information sources, start with your doctor or one of the organizations listed below:

> **American Cancer Society**
> National Headquarters
> 1599 Clifton Road N.E.
> Atlanta, GA 30329
> (800)227-2345
> www.cancer.org

American Foundation for Urologic Disease
1128 N. Charles St.
Baltimore, MD 21201
(800)242-2383
www.afud.org

Provides referrals to local urologists and general information on urinary-tract problems.

Cancer Information Service
(800)422-6237

These are cancer-information specialists. They can provide free brochures on nutrition, metastasis, regional support organizations, prostate-cancer research, and radiation therapies—among dozens of others. Trained counselors can also tell you about clinical trials for prostate cancer, performed through the National Cancer Institute.

Impotents Anonymous
P.O. Box 5299
Marysyille, TN 37802
(615)983-6064

Founded by diabetic impotence patient Bruce MacKenzie, this group helps the chronically impotent man regain his self-confidence and explore his options.

Local Hospital Support Programs

Most hospitals with cancer-treatment units also provide patient-support groups, educational seminars, and informational meetings. Contact the social-services department of your hospital or ask your doctor for a referral.

National Cancer Institute
Building 82, Room 123
Bethesda, MD 20892
(800)422-6237
www.nci.nih.gov

This federal institute offers a periodical prostate cancer research update. It can usually inform you about clinical trials that are taking place in your area.

National Council Against Health Fraud
P.O. Box 141
Fort Lee, NJ 07024
(201)723-2955
www.ncahf.org

This nonprofit group provides information on health frauds, quack cures, and misinformation in public-health systems. It produces a brochure on a lineup of "questionable" cancer cures. Some users, however, feel the group is unfairly biased toward medical and surgical treatments.

National Institute of Diabetes, Digestive and Kidney Diseases
part of the National Institutes of Health
Bethesda, MD 20892
(301)496-3583
www.niddk.nih.gov

Referrals are usually available to local clinical trials in experimental treatments for BPH and prostatitis.

National Second Surgical Opinion Program Hotline
(800)237-4666

Call this toll-free number for free information on urinary incontinence.

Physicians Data Query (PDQ) at the National Cancer Institute

This is a data base for up-to-date cancer-treatment information. It is regularly updated and approved by cancer researchers. Have your doctor call the PDQ or use your own FAX access. For a six-or-more-page FAX update about prostate cancer and its treatment options, call (301)402-5874. When instructed, enter the prostate cancer patient information code: 201229.

Wellness Community
35 E. Seventh St., Suite 412
Cincinnati, OH 45202
(888)793-9355, fax (513)421-7119
www.wellness-community.org

This is a nonprofit organization that provides a range of support services to cancer patients and their families in comfortable home-like settings free of charge.

- APPENDIX II •

Bibliography

The author owes a debt of gratitude to many experts, journals, authors, and health-care workers who were generous with their time and knowledge. A few of the works used as reference for this volume are listed below:

Bricklin, Mark. *The Practical Encyclopedia of Natural Healing*, revised edition. New York, Penguin Books, 1990

Cunningham, Chet. *The Prostate Problem*. New York, Windsor-Pinnacle Books, 1990

Dunn, Lavon 3., Nutrition Almanac, Third Edition. New York, McGraw-Hill Publishing Co. 1990.

Editors, et. al., *Bircher-Bender Handout far Manner mit Prostataleiden*. Bircher-Benner-Verlag GmbH, Bad Homburg, Germany, 1992

Ethical Nutrients Corp., *Nutritional Research News*, issue 9

Hoffman, Matthew and William LeGro. *Disease Free: How to Prevent, Treat and Cure More Than 150 Illnesses and Conditions*. Pennsylvania; Rodale Press, 1993

Hylton, William H., ed. *The Rodale Herb Book*. Emmaus, Pennsylvania, Rodale Press, 1974

Kordel, Lelord. *Natural Folk Remedies*. New York: G.P.

Putnam's Sons, 1974

Matsen, Jonn, M.D. *The Mysterious Cause of lliness: How to Overcome Every Disease from Constipation to Cancer.* Canfield, Ohio, Fischer Publishing Co., 1988

What Every Man Should Know About His Prostate and A Patient Guide: Proscar., Merck Pharmaceutical, Chapel Hill, North Carolina, 1993

Pschyrembel Klinisches Worterbuch. DeGruyter: 1986 Berlin, Germany

"The Killer We Don't Discuss" and *"To Test or Not to Test,"* articles in *Newsweek* magazine, volume 122, no. 26, Dec.27, 1993, pp 40-43

Rossman, Isadore, M.D., *Looking Forward.*, E.P. Dutton, 1989

Rossman, Isadore, M.D., *The Best Treatment.*, Bantam, 1992

Rous, Stephen N., M.D., *The Prostate Book*: updated edition., New York: W.W. Norton, 1992

Shapiro, Charles E., M.D., and Kathleen Doheny. *The Well Informed Patient's Guide to Prostate Problems.* New York, Dell Publishing, 1993

Simons, Anne, M.D., Bobbie Hasselbring and Michael Castleman. *Before You Call the Doctor.* New York, Fawcett Columbine, 1992

Stoltz, Craig. "Prostate cancer: a Bipartisan Issue". *USA weekend magazine.* Dec. 3-5 edition, 1993

Treben, Maria. *Healing Through God's Pharmacy: Advice and Experiences With Medicinal Herbs.* Steyr, Austria: Wilhelm Ennsthaler, 1993

Treben, Maria. *Maria Treben's Cures.* Steyr, Austria, Wilhelm Ennsthaler, 1980

Index

NOTES

NOTES

NOTES